Childhood Depression

About the Author

Martha C. Tompson, PhD, is a licensed clinical psychologist in Massachusetts. She has been a faculty member in the Department of Psychological and Brain Sciences at Boston University for over 25 years and is the Director of Clinical Training for the Doctoral Program in Clinical Psychology. Dr. Tompson has spent her career developing and evaluating family-based treatment for mental health problems in children and adults. She lives in the Boston area with her husband and has two grown children.

Advances in Psychotherapy – Evidence-Based Practice

Series Editor
Danny Wedding, PhD, MPH, Professor Emeritus, University of Missouri–Saint Louis, MO

Associate Editors
Jonathan S. Comer, PhD, Professor of Psychology and Psychiatry, Director of Mental Health Interventions and Technology (MINT) Program, Center for Children and Families, Florida International University, Miami, FL

J. Kim Penberthy, PhD, ABPP, Professor of Psychiatry & Neurobehavioral Sciences, University of Virginia, Charlottesville, VA

Kenneth E. Freedland, PhD, Professor of Psychiatry and Psychology, Washington University School of Medicine, St. Louis, MO

Linda C. Sobell, PhD, ABPP, Professor, Center for Psychological Studies, Nova Southeastern University, Ft. Lauderdale, FL

The basic objective of this series is to provide therapists with practical, evidence-based treatment guidance for the most common disorders seen in clinical practice – and to do so in a reader-friendly manner. Each book in the series is both a compact "how-to" reference on a particular disorder for use by professional clinicians in their daily work and an ideal educational resource for students as well as for practice-oriented continuing education.

The most important feature of the books is that they are practical and easy to use: All are structured similarly and all provide a compact and easy-to-follow guide to all aspects that are relevant in real-life practice. Tables, boxed clinical "pearls," marginal notes, and summary boxes assist orientation, while checklists provide tools for use in daily practice.

Continuing Education Credits

Psychologists and other healthcare providers may earn five continuing education credits for reading the books in the *Advances in Psychotherapy* series and taking a multiple-choice exam. This continuing education program is a partnership of Hogrefe Publishing and the National Register of Health Service Psychologists. Details are available at https://www.hogrefe.com/us/cenatreg

The National Register of Health Service Psychologists is approved by the American Psychological Association to sponsor continuing education for psychologists. The National Register maintains responsibility for this program and its content.

Advances in Psychotherapy – Evidence-Based Practice, Volume 54

Childhood Depression

Martha C. Tompson
Department of Psychological and Brain Sciences, Boston University, MA

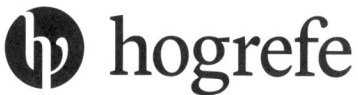

Library of Congress of Congress Cataloging in Publication information for the print version of this book is available via the Library of Congress Marc Database under the Library of Congress Control Number 2024935167

Library and Archives Canada Cataloguing in Publication
Title: Childhood depression / Martha C. Tompson, Department of Psychological and Brain Sciences, Boston University, MA.
Names: Tompson, Martha C., author.
Series: Advances in psychotherapy--evidence-based practice ; v. 54.
Description: Series statement: Advances in psychotherapy--evidence-based practice ; volume 54 | Includes bibliographical references.
Identifiers: Canadiana (print) 20240343336 | Canadiana (ebook) 20240343360 | ISBN 9780889375185 (softcover) | ISBN 9781613345184 (EPUB) | ISBN 9781616765187 (PDF)
Subjects: LCSH: Depression in children. | LCSH: Depression in children—Diagnosis. | LCSH: Depression in children—Treatment. | LCSH: Child psychotherapy. | LCSH: Family psychotherapy. | LCSH: Cognitive therapy.
Classification: LCC RJ506.D4 T66 2024 | DDC 150 | 618.92/8527—dc23

© 2025 by Hogrefe Publishing
www.hogrefe.com

The authors and publisher have made every effort to ensure that the information contained in this text is in accord with the current state of scientific knowledge, recommendations, and practice at the time of publication. In spite of this diligence, errors cannot be completely excluded. Also, due to changing regulations and continuing research, information may become outdated at any point. The authors and publisher disclaim any responsibility for any consequences which may follow from the use of information presented in this book.

Registered trademarks are not noted specifically as such in this publication. The use of descriptive names, registered names, and trademarks does not imply, even in the absence of a specific statement, that such names are exempt from the relevant protective laws and regulations and therefore free for general use.

The cover image is an agency photo depicting models. Use of the photo on this publication does not imply any connection between the content of this publication and any person depicted in the cover image.
Cover image: © Solovyova – iStock.com

PUBLISHING OFFICES
USA: Hogrefe Publishing Corporation, 44 Merrimac St., Newburyport, MA 01950
Phone 978 255 3700; E-mail customersupport@hogrefe.com
EUROPE: Hogrefe Publishing GmbH, Merkelstr. 3, 37085 Göttingen, Germany
Phone +49 551 99950 0, Fax +49 551 99950 111; E-mail publishing@hogrefe.com

SALES & DISTRIBUTION
USA: Hogrefe Publishing, Customer Services Department,
30 Amberwood Parkway, Ashland, OH 44805
Phone 800 228 3749, Fax 419 281 6883; E-mail customersupport@hogrefe.com
UK: Hogrefe Publishing, c/o Marston Book Services Ltd., 160 Eastern Ave.,
Milton Park, Abingdon, OX14 4SB
Phone +44 1235 465577, Fax +44 1235 465556; E-mail direct.orders@marston.co.uk
EUROPE: Hogrefe Publishing, Merkelstr. 3, 37085 Göttingen, Germany
Phone +49 551 99950 0, Fax +49 551 99950 111; E-mail publishing@hogrefe.com

OTHER OFFICES
CANADA: Hogrefe Publishing Corporation, 82 Laird Drive, East York, Ontario, M4G 3V1
SWITZERLAND: Hogrefe Publishing, Länggass-Strasse 76, 3012 Bern

No part of this book may be reproduced, stored in a retrieval system or transmitted, in any form or by any means, electronic, mechanical, photocopying, microfilming, recording or otherwise, without written permission from the publisher.

Printed and bound in the USA

ISBN 978-0-88937-518-5 (print) · ISBN 978-1-61676-518-7 (PDF) · ISBN 978-1-61334-518-4 (EPUB)
https://doi.org/10.1027/00518-000

Contents

Preface		vii
1	**History**	1
1.1	Diagnostic Criteria and Description	1
1.1.1	Major Depressive Disorder	2
1.1.2	Persistent Depressive Disorder	3
1.1.3	Disruptive Mood Dysregulation Disorder	3
1.1.4	Adjustment Disorders	4
1.1.5	Other Depressive Disorders	4
1.2	Epidemiology	5
1.3	Course and Prognosis	9
1.4	Differential Diagnosis	10
1.5	Comorbidities	10
1.6	Issues Gaining Increased Attention	10
2	**Theories and Contributing Factors**	12
2.1.	Biological Contributors	12
2.1.1	Neural Factors	12
2.1.2	Endocrine-Related and HPA Axis	13
2.1.3	Genetic Factors and Parental Depression	14
2.2	Child and Developmental Risk Factors	15
2.2.1	Developmental Risk	15
2.2.2	Temperament/Personality	16
2.2.3	Cognitive Contributors	17
2.2.4	Earlier Mental Health Problems	18
2.3	Environmental and Psychosocial Risk Factors	18
2.3.1	Stress Context	18
2.3.2	Family Functioning	19
2.3.3	Peer Stress	20
2.4	Models/Theories	21
2.4.1	Vulnerability–Stress Models	21
2.4.2	Cognitive-Behavioral Models	21
2.4.3	Interpersonal and Stress-Generation Models	21
2.5	An Integrative Model to Guide Treatment	22
3	**Evaluation**	25
3.1	Reporters	25
3.2	Special Considerations in Evaluation	26
3.3	Diagnostic Tools	28
3.3.1	Depression Screening	28
3.3.2	Diagnostic Interviews	29

3.3.3	Depression Symptom Rating Scales	31
3.3.4	Observational and Technological Approaches	33
3.3.5	Tools for Evaluating Suicidal Thoughts and Behaviors	34
4	**Treatment: A Family-Based Approach**	**35**
4.1	Evidence Base for Child and Adolescent Depression Treatment	35
4.1.1	Psychosocial Interventions	35
4.1.2	Medication Interventions	36
4.2	Family-Focused Treatment for Childhood Depression (FFT-CD)	37
4.2.1	Structure of the Therapy	38
4.2.2	Important Treatment Strategies	41
4.2.3	Setting the Stage with Individual Sessions	42
4.2.4	Family Sessions	47
4.3	Challenges in Implementing FFT-CD	68
4.4	Efficacy of FFT-CD	70
5	**Case Vignettes**	**74**
6	**Further Reading**	**85**
7	**References**	**86**
8	**Appendix: Tools and Resources**	**99**

Preface

The past decade has witnessed a dramatic 33% growth of major depressive disorder (MDD) in adolescents (Blue Cross Blue Shield, 2018) and a startling 100% increase in emergency room visits for attempted suicides, self-injury, or suicidal ideation (Mercado et al., 2017). With 1–2% of primary school-aged youth suffering from MDD and another 0.6–1.7% from persistent depressive (dysthymic) disorder, childhood-onset depressive disorders are significantly less common than adolescent-onset forms (Birmaher et al., 2007). However, onset in childhood is associated with significant morbidity and significant interference in the crucial developmental tasks that present during middle childhood.

Youth depression unfolds within a developmental and systems context and integration of families into treatment has a number of advantages. From a developmental standpoint, many therapy approaches for depression do not adequately consider developmental limitations during middle to late childhood. For example, cognitive behavioral therapy (CBT) approaches assume that negative/maladaptive ways of attending to, processing, and remembering contribute to individual vulnerability to depression (Beck & Bredemeier, 2016); however, this approach does not always fit well with the cognitive-developmental capabilities of preadolescent children. The ability to use higher-order generalizations to understand oneself and others emerges gradually across childhood and the kinds of cognitive vulnerabilities emphasized in cognitive therapy for adolescents and adults may not yet be stable (Garber & Flynn, 2001). From a systems standpoint, compared to adults and adolescents, preadolescents are more strongly embedded in their family context and thus engagement of families in treatment is particularly helpful. Parents provide support and feedback throughout this period, interface with the community settings (communicating with schools, attending churches, setting up extracurricular activities) and social relationships (setting up playdates, transporting children to social activities), and model/teach coping and other key life skills. Thus, it is unlikely that treatments that work well for adolescents and adults can simply be extended downward; children may need a more developmentally informed treatment approach.

In this book we present family-focused treatment for childhood depression (FFT-CD), which was designed specifically to address the developmental needs of school-aged children and their parents. The emphasis is on fostering positive and supportive parent–child interactions that scaffold the development of a positive self, helping parents provide the child additional positive feedback on their developmentally appropriate achievements, and enhancing family and child coping. Through providing a background on childhood depression, giving a step-by-step description of this intervention approach, and illustrating its implementation with case examples, we hope to enhance work with depressed children and strengthen their families to move forward.

1

History

Prior to the early 1980s depressive disorders were not regularly diagnosed in youth. Psychodynamic approaches viewed children as incapable of experiencing adult-like depression due to inadequate super-ego development (Mahler, 1961). Another dominant view was that children displayed other syndromes, such as externalizing symptoms, as a means of expressing their dysphoria – a masked depression. However, in 1980 Carlson and Cantwell published a seminal article, titled "Unmasking Masked Depression," in which they applied adult diagnostic criteria to youth and found they could reliably diagnose depression, particularly when using a systematic interview, and that children with other masked symptoms (e.g., conduct, anorexia) did not necessarily meet criteria for depression. Decades of careful research followed to evaluate the diagnostic reliability, risk factors, course, family aggregation, associated psychosocial circumstances and features, and treatment of youth depression.

> Depressive disorders can be reliably diagnosed in youth

1.1 Diagnostic Criteria and Description

In this section, we discuss some of the basic terms, categories, and criteria for describing and diagnosing depressive disorders in youth that are described in the *Diagnostic and Statistical Manual of Mental Disorders* (5th ed.; *DSM-5*; American Psychiatric Association [APA], 2013) and the *ICD-10 Classification of Mental and Behavioural Disorders: Diagnostic Criteria for Research* (World Health Organization, 1993) – two of the most widely used classification systems. Table 1 provides the categories of depressive disorders that are listed in the two systems.

> Diagnosed with the DSM-5 and the ICD-10

Although there are differences in the symptoms listed in these two classification systems, depressive disorder categories and symptoms are highly overlapping. Importantly, for most of these disorders, children and adolescents are diagnosed using the same diagnostic criteria used to diagnose depressive disorders in adults.

> Other diagnostic considerations include adjustment disorder with mixed anxiety and depressed mood

Both systems include, under mood disorders, diagnoses of major depressive disorder (MDD), disruptive mood dysregulation disorder, premenstrual dysphoric disorder, and depression secondary to a medical condition or to a medication/substance. There are also categories for specified and unspecified depressive disorders. Additional relevant diagnoses are included under

Table 1
Overlapping Diagnostic Categories and Codes for Depressive Disorders in *DSM-5* and *ICD-10*

Diagnosis	DSM-5	ICD-10
Major depressive disorder		
Single episode	296.2	F32
Recurrent episode	296.3W	F33
Persistent depressive disorder	300.4	F34.1
Disruptive mood dysregulation disorder	296.99	F31.81
Premenstrual dysphoric disorder	635.4	F32.81
Depression secondary to a medical condition	293.83	F06.3x
Depression secondary to a medication/substance	291.89 (alcohol) 292.8x (substance specifier)	F10–F19
Specified depressive disorder	311	F32.89
Unspecified depressive disorder	311	F32.9
Adjustment disorder with depressed mood	309.00	F43.21
Adjustment disorder with mixed anxiety and depressed mood	309.28	F43.23

adjustment disorders, including adjustment disorder with depressed mood and adjustment disorder with mixed anxiety and depressed mood, as these are frequent presentations of depression in youth. To enhance readability, and given the high overlap between these two systems, we focus on *DSM-5* diagnostic categories and criteria throughout this volume. Descriptions of some of the most commonly encountered depressive disorders in youth are included below.

1.1.1 Major Depressive Disorder

> MDD includes depressed or irritable mood, diminished interests, fatigue, and impacts on memory, appetite, and sleep

MDD is the most commonly diagnosed depressive disorder in adults and children. Over the years it has frequently been referred to as the common cold of psychological disorders but its impact is far more serious. A diagnosis of MDD requires at least a 2-week duration with five of the following symptoms occurring most days for most of the day with at least one of the first two being present: depressed mood, significant loss of interest and/or pleasure in activities, weight loss/diminished appetite, sleep disturbance, psychomotor disturbance, fatigue/loss of energy, feelings of worthlessness or excessive guilt, impaired concentration or indecisiveness, and recurrent thoughts of death or suicidal thoughts or behaviors. For youth, mood may be irritable – a frequent parental experience. In addition to these primary symptoms are a plethora of associated symptoms, such as hopelessness, pessimism, and helplessness.

MDD should not be diagnosed if symptoms are due to the impact of a substance or a medical condition, are better explained by another disorder (e.g., psychotic), or if there is a history of mania or hypomania. Specifier codes are used to delineate episode type (single episode or recurrent), severity (mild, moderate, severe, with psychotic features), course (full or partial remission), and accompanying features (anxious distress, mixed features, melancholia, atypical, types of psychotic feature, catatonia, seasonal pattern). For MDD to be considered recurrent there must be at least 2 months between episodes in which diagnostic criteria are not met. Given the wide range of potential severity of MDD, it is essential to have a complete evaluation of symptoms and measures of severity and impairment in diagnosing it.

> MDD evaluation includes episode type and recurrence, severity, temporal course, and impairment

1.1.2 Persistent Depressive Disorder

Persistent depressive disorder (PDD, *DSM-5*) combines previous *DSM* diagnoses of chronic MDD and dysthymic disorder/dysthymia. Dysthymic disorder in *DSM-IV-TR* (American Psychiatric Association, 2000) and dysthymia in *DSM-III-R* (American Psychiatric Association, 1987) described a low level but highly protracted depressive disorder. The PDD diagnosis acknowledges the reality that symptoms of depression can wax and wane – both in adults and children. Low level depressions can worsen into full MDD episodes, and recovery from a full episode can be only partial. Children with this presentation were described as having double depression – a major depressive episode superimposed on a longer dysthymic pattern. To meet criteria for PDD, youth much experience depressed mood most of the day, most days for at least a year, accompanied by at least two of the following symptoms – changes in appetite (poor appetite or overeating), problems with sleep (insomnia or hypersomnia), low energy level or fatigue, low self-esteem, poor concentration or problems with decision-making, and hopelessness. The youth with PDD is never without symptoms for as long as two months during the year. Similar to MDD it has a number of specifiers for accompanying features, severity (mild, moderate, severe), remission, and course (pure dysthymic, persistent major depressive, intermittent major depressive). All childhood and adolescent depressions would be considered early onset (prior to age 21).

1.1.3 Disruptive Mood Dysregulation Disorder

This disorder is characterized by severe temper outbursts that recur at least three times weekly over a year or more and are markedly more intense or lengthy than would be expected either developmentally or based on circumstances or environmental triggers. The outbursts occur in at least two settings (i.e., home, school, with peers), and the mood between outbursts

> DMDD includes intense and frequent emotional outbursts, and chronic irritability

is frequently angry/irritable to a degree that is noted by others in the environment (i.e., parents, siblings, teachers, peers). For a diagnosis to be made, symptoms of this disorder must emerge prior to age 10. Children with disruptive mood dysregulation disorder cannot also be simultaneously diagnosed with bipolar disorder, intermittent explosive disorder, or oppositional defiant disorder. However, this disorder can co-occur with MDD, attention deficit hyperactivity disorder (ADHD), and conduct and substance use disorders. Disruptive mood dysregulation disorder is new in the *DSM-5*, and research here lags behind other mood disorders. There are not clear diagnostic criteria for this disorder in the *ICD-10*.

1.1.4 Adjustment Disorders

Adjustment disorders develop in response to identifiable stressful events and emerge within 3 months of their occurrence. The symptoms are out of proportion to the stressful events, even considering contextual and cultural factors that might impact the circumstances, and are associated with significant impairment in functioning. Adjustment disorder with depressed mood is characterized by low mood, crying, and hopelessness but may have other symptoms as well. In adjustment disorder with mixed anxiety and depression we also see worry, nervousness, and separation concerns with the depressed symptoms. While impaired, youth with adjustment disorders do not meet full criteria for MDD. The adjustment disorder symptoms tend not to last beyond 6 months after the stressful circumstances have resolved. However, the timing can be challenging in diagnosing adjustment disorders in youth, as some stressful triggers are one-time events (e.g., automobile accident) and others are complex stressors that can lead to multiple life changes/challenges (e.g., parental separation and divorce); thus, timing when the event resolves is not always straightforward.

In extensive research examining the natural history and characteristics of youth depressive disorders, Kovacs and colleagues (1984a, b) found that adjustment disorders do not cluster with MDD and PDD. Adjustment disorders demonstrated a much greater likelihood of recovery and low likelihood of subsequent MDD episodes. MDD and dysthymia frequently overlapped, and dysthymia was a predictor of subsequent MDD. In contrast, adjustment disorder with depressed mood did not predict future MDD episodes. Thus, MDD and *DSM-5* PDD appear to represent a broader depression-spectrum phenomenon; whereas adjustment disorder with depressed mood appears to be a distinct, reactive, circumstantial problem.

> Adjustment disorders are distinct, reactive, circumstantial problems

1.1.5 Other Depressive Disorders

There may be other nonspecified depressive disorders that are experienced across the lifespan, including by children and adolescents. These may include recurrent brief depression, short-duration depression, and depression with insufficient symptoms. The latter may be particularly important given the challenges inherent in evaluating symptoms in younger children in particular.

1.2 Epidemiology

Studies on the epidemiology of depressive disorders in youth have been conducted in numerous countries. Table 2 outlines findings from selected studies for MDD, as few studies have examined the epidemiology of other depressive disorders. Studies used different strategies for examining the epidemiology of depressive disorders across development. First, they used different periods of assessment – point prevalence (how many meet criteria for a depressive disorder at the time of assessment), 3 months, 6 months, 12 months, lifetime. Second, as studies were done at different times, they used different diagnostic criteria – *DSM-III* (American Psychiatric Association, 1980), *DSM-IIIR*, *DSM-IV* (American Psychiatric Association, 1994). Third, they used different age groupings – individual ages, combining across ages. All of these differences make it more challenging to draw firm conclusions. Although there are clearly differences in the rates of depressive disorders in youth by age, there is far less data on preschoolers and children than adolescents. Preschool onset of depression has rarely been studied and with only small samples. These suggest very low rates of depression in this age group. Some studies have found higher rates but these have been conducted with high-risk samples of children with depressed parents and likely heavy genetic loading for mood disorders. It may be that depression is rare for very young children outside of more high-risk contexts. A few more studies across a range of countries have been conducted with school-aged youth (ages 7–12 years) with 12-month prevalence estimated between 3% and 6% for MDD. Adolescent depression is much more common with epidemiologic studies with a 12-month prevalence of up to 20% for MDD or other depressive disorders.

There also may be gender differences in the risk of depression across development. In addition to their greater prevalence, adolescent-onset depressive disorders appear to differ from childhood-onset disorders in their gender distribution. Like adult-onset depression, adolescent-onset depression is much more likely to occur in women/girls than in men/boys. Over two decades ago Hankin and colleagues (1998) observed in a large dataset that, although rates of depression were similar between boys and girls before age 13 years, around age 13 rates for girls began to increase. By age 15 rates for both boys and girls were increasing but rates for girls were doing so at a much steeper rate leading to a significant gender gap. Another study indicated that this increase in risk for girls only emerged when they were midway through puberty (Angold et al., 1998). A more recent meta-analysis of numerous studies on the gender distribution of depressive disorders (Salk et al., 2017) indicated that by age 12 there is already an approximately 2:1 ratio of girls to boys, that the ratio increases to an almost 3:1 ratio by late adolescence: By

> Depression appears to be rare for very young children outside of high-risk contexts

> Risk of depression for girls has a steeper rise than the risk for boys after puberty

Table 2
Prevalence of Depressive Disorders in Youth From Selected US and International Studies

Study	DSM	Time frame	N	Age	% MDD	Country
Anderson et al. (1987)	III	12 months	792	11	1.8	New Zealand
Angold et al. (1998)	IV	3 months	970	10–14	3.1	USA
	IV	3 months	928	11–15	3.2	USA
	IV	3 months	820	12–16	2.7	USA
Bird et al. (1993)	III	6 months	222	9–16	8.0	USA
Canino et al. (2004)	IV	12 months	1,886	4–17	MDD 3.0 DYS 0.5	Puerto Rico
Costello et al. (2003)	IV	3 months	936	9–10	0.5	USA
	IV	3 months	901	11	1.9	USA
	IV	3 months	854	12	0.4	USA
	IV	3 months	833	13	2.6	USA
	IV	3 months	913	14	2.7	USA
	IV	3 months	1,136	15	3.7	USA
	IV	3 months	1,101	16	3.1	USA
Frost et al. (1989)	III	12 months	850	13	2.2	New Zealand
Kashani et al. (1983)	III	Current	641	9	MDD 1.8 Minor 2.5	New Zealand
Kashani et al. (1986)[1]	III	Current	109	2.5–6	MDD 1.8 DD 6.4	USA
Kashani et al. (1987)	III	Current	150	14–16	MDD 4.7 DYS 3.3	USA
Kinyanda et al. (2013)	IV	Current	286	<5	2.8	Uganda
	IV	Current	416	6–9	5.8	Uganda
	IV	Current	550	10–13	11.1	Uganda
	IV	Current	335	14–19	12.8	Uganda
Lewinsohn et al. (1993)	III-R	Point lifetime	1,710	14–18	MDD 2.57 DYS 0.53 MDD 18.48 DYS 3.22	USA
McGee et al. (1990)	III	12 months	943	15	4.2	New Zealand
Mohammadi et al. (2019)[2]	IV	Lifetime	9,741	6–9	0.7	Iran
		Lifetime	10,028	10–14	1.6	Iran
		Lifetime	8,842	15–18	3.3	Iran

Table 2 Continued						
Study	DSM	Time frame	N	Age	% MDD	Country
Olsson & von Knorring (1999)	III-R	1 year	2,300	16–17	5.8	Sweden
	III-R	Lifetime	2,300	16–17	11.4	Sweden
Reinherz et al. (1993)	III-R	6 months	386	18	6.0	USA
Sawyer et al (2018)	IV	12 months	5,359	6–17	3.2	Australia
Shaffer et al. (1996)	III-R	6 months	1,285	9–17	Mild 6.2 Moderate 4.5 Severe 2.5	USA
Simonoff et al. (1997)	III-R	3 months	2,762	8–16	1.2	USA
Velez et al. (1989)	IIIR	12 months	776	9–18	3.4	USA
Wichstrøm et al. (2012)	IV	3 months	995	4	2.0	Norway

Note. MDD = major depressive disorder; DD = dysthymic disorder; DYS = dysthymia. [1] Depression was evaluated using depression symptom checklist. [2] Major depressive disorder or other depressive disorder including "depressive episodes lasting at least 6 months but with three to four symptoms, or depressive episodes with five or more symptoms that lasted 1–2 weeks."

the early 20s and beyond the ratio was somewhat lower at approximately 2:1 but still significantly skewed toward women. As noted previously, there are far fewer studies of children younger than 12, and thus these younger age groups were not considered in this meta-analysis. However, other studies suggest an almost even ratio of girls to boys prior to age 12 with a possible slight overrepresentation of boys (Hankin et al., 1998; Angold et al., 1998). Thus, it is not entirely clear when the gender risk changes. Numerous contributing factors have been marshalled to explain the emergence of this gender difference, including hormones, changing social roles, gender differences in life stress, and physical changes in girls that lead to increased body dissatisfaction. Examination of depression in sexual minority youth has become a topic of significant interest in the past decade and prevalence appears high in these youth, particularly during the stressful time when they question their identity (Guz et al., 2021).

A few studies in the US have examined racial/ethnic group differences in prevalence of youth depressive disorders. This is a challenging literature to unpack, as racial/ethnic group has been aggregated differently across studies, and, depending on where the study was conducted, only some racial/ethnic groups are well represented in samples. The vast majority of studies do not disaggregate by age, gender, and ethnicity simultaneously, making it difficult to discern potentially complex patterns. In addition, studies use different measures, with some evaluating symptoms and others assessing disorders. The lack of availability of adequate studies precludes evaluation of these differences in preschool and school-aged youth; however, it does appear that the greater preponderance of depression in adolescent girls compared to adolescent boys is seen across racial/ethnic groups. Several studies suggest that Hispanic/Latinx youth may experience more depressive symptoms (Roberts & Chen, 1995) and disorders (Roberts et al., 1997) than other racial/ethnic groups. Other studies have found that Hispanic/Latina girls are at particularly high risk (McLaughlin et al., 2007). Recent studies have underscored the increased risk for high depressive symptoms and suicidal ideation and behaviors in Native Hawaiian/Pacific Islander, Native American/Alaskan, and multiracial youth compared to other groups of adolescents (Wyatt et al., 2015). Interestingly, among the rural participants in the Great Smoky Mountains study, Anglo youth were significantly more likely than African American youth to report 3-month prevalence for both major and minor depression but not dysthymia (Angold et al., 2002). There are likely numerous causal factors that may explain differences in rates of depressive symptoms and disorders between racial/ethnic groups, including differences in socioeconomic status (SES), access to community resources, immigration stress, community and family cohesion and support, and experiences with discrimination, as well as others.

Suicidal ideation and behavior (e.g., attempts, completed suicide) is a risk among depressed youth

Suicidal ideation and behavior are frequent concomitants of depressive disorder. Although suicide certainly is not limited to those with depressive disorders, upward of 60% of youth are depressed at the time of completed suicide, and depression is a powerful risk factor (Cash & Bridge, 2009). Suicide is the second leading cause of death among those 10–14 year of age and the third leading cause of death among those 15–24 years of age. Suicide completion risk increases across youth development with rates low during childhood and exploding during the adolescent years. Among adolescents we see stark differences in rates of completed suicide by gender with boys/young men being *higher* than girls/young women (22.7 vs. 5.8 per 100,000; National Institute of Mental Health, 2022); however, we see more than twice the number of suicide attempts in 12–17-year-old girls/women compared to 12–17-year-old boys/young men (Yard et al., 2021). This apparent contradiction appears to be accounted for by the means of suicide being different across genders, with boys more likely to use more lethal means (firearms and hanging) than girls (Miranda-Mendizabal et al., 2019). There are complex relationships between suicide and race/ethnicity. Native American youth appear to have the highest rates of completed suicide, followed by non-Hispanic White youth; however, Black youth, particularly boys, appear to have demonstrated increased rates in the past decade. To further complicate matters, there are notable differences in ethnic groups in different indicators of suicidality – ideation, attempts, and completed suicide. There is some evidence that the gender difference in suicide risk is narrowing in the US in the last few decades for all racial and ethnic groups (Ruch et al., 2019). Both depression and suicide appear particularly elevated among youth questioning their sexual orientation and/or gender identity (Guz et al., 2021).

Minority stress factors increase risk for ethnic/racial and sexual minority youth

1.3 Course and Prognosis

The course of depressive disorders in youth is variable, and the data are mixed as to whether or not childhood-onset and adolescent-onset disorders are similar in their outcome (Birmaher et al., 2004). Although depression during childhood may be associated with longer episodes, depression during adolescence shows comparatively greater risk for suicide. Overall, depression occurring first in childhood and adolescence appears to be associated with greater comorbidity, worse functioning, and more episodes and suicide attempts than depression first occurring in adulthood (Zisook et al., 2007). Given the focus of this volume on the treatment of childhood depressive disorders, the remainder of this chapter and beyond will focus on this early onset, primarily prepubertal depression.

By a number of indicators, depressive disorders in childhood are associated with significant morbidity. First, children with depressive disorders show high chronicity and severity. Although they can be diagnosed after only 2 weeks of symptoms, untreated MDD episodes last on average 7 to 9 months (McCauley et al., 1993). In these early studies dysthymic disorder tends to have an earlier onset in childhood than does MDD. In terms of chronicity, although PDD/dysthymic disorder can be diagnosed after a year of ongoing symptoms in youth, compared to 2 years in adults, it has been found to persist significantly longer than 1 year; longitudinal data suggest a typical length of approximately 4 years. Although this diagnosis was intended to characterize those low level depressions that, while less severe than MDD, were chronic in nature, youth who met criteria for dysthymia are at significantly enhanced risk for an eventual MDD episode (Kovacs et al., 1994). Second, children with depressive disorders have a high risk of relapse and bipolar outcome. In the 5 years following an MDD episode, 70% of youth were found to have a relapse (Kovacs, 1996). In a 15-year naturalistic follow-up of MDD children, 12% showed manic "switching" and met diagnostic criteria for bipolar I disorder; another 14% met criteria for bipolar II disorder (Kovacs et al., 2016). Third, children with depressive disorders are at increased longer term risk of suicide. Following depressed youth for an average of approximately 12 years, Weissman and colleagues (1999) found 27% had a history of suicide attempts with approximately one third happening during the prepubertal period. Fourth, children with depression show significant social impairment during episodes, and these do not appear to remit even following symptom improvement (Puig-Antich et al., 1985a, 1985b). This appears particularly true of dysthymic disorders, as the sheer chronicity of these syndromes lead to powerful negative impacts on social functioning in children lasting well beyond the symptoms themselves. Overall, early onset depression, when untreated or ineffectively treated, is predictive of chronic problems during adolescence as well as adult depression (Weissman et al., 1999).

> Depression in childhood is often severe, chronic, and recurrent

1.4 Differential Diagnosis

In diagnosing depressive disorders, several differential diagnoses should be considered and ruled out. First, for youth with a history of manic and/or hypomanic symptoms, bipolar disorders – bipolar I, bipolar II, bipolar not otherwise specified (NOS), cyclothymia – would be diagnosed. Second, when symptoms occur only due to a general medical condition or a medication or other drug, a diagnosis of depressive disorder should not be made. Medical consultation should be a regular part of evaluation for depressive disorders. Third, although depressive disorders can occur with anxiety disorder and ADHD, it is important not to overdiagnose. The distractibility, concentration difficulties, and irritability that are seen in depressive disorder can also occur in youth with ADHD and anxiety disorders. These disorders should be carefully ruled out or evaluated as comorbid conditions. Finally, the distinction between MDD and adjustment disorders is crucial, as there are important implications for course, as detailed above. Although both disorders can be preceded and triggered by a stressful life event or circumstances, adjustment disorders do not meet full MDD criteria.

1.5 Comorbidities

Depression has high psychiatric comorbidity

Depressive disorders in youth are frequently comorbid with other psychiatric and medical conditions. Approximately 40–70% of depressed youth have at least one comorbid disorder (Birmaher et al., 1996); in most cases the comorbidities preceded the onset of depression. The most common psychiatric comorbidities are apparent in both childhood- and adolescent-onset depressive disorders and include anxiety, ADHD, and substance use (Rohde et al., 2013). Importantly, comorbidity appears in both clinical samples (e.g., Kovacs, 1996) and community samples (e.g., Angold & Costello, 1993), suggesting that it is not just an artifact of more severe, referred cases that tend to be seen in clinical settings. In terms of medical comorbidities, chronic medical disease including asthma, inflammatory bowel disease/recurrent abdominal pain, and sickle cell anemia, may increase risk for depressive symptoms and disorders than diabetes, cancer, and cystic fibrosis. Interestingly, within samples of each chronic disease group there appears to be a high degree of variability of depressive symptoms that is not accounted for by illness severity or duration (Bennett, 1994).

1.6 Issues Gaining Increased Attention

In the last decade, new considerations have emerged as we strive to understand the landscape of youth depressive disorders. Two in particular are highlighted here: apparent increases in rates of depressive disorders and the inadequate availability of treatment, particularly for ethnic and racial minority youth.

Across the last decade, there appears to be a substantial increase in the rate of depressive disorders in youth. The Federal Interagency Forum on Child and Family Statistics published a report – *America's Children in Brief: Key National Indicators of Well-Being, 2023* – that provides statistics on children's health. These data reflect an increase in the prevalence of major depressive episodes over the last couple of decades for all ages between 12 and 17 years. There is little data available to shed light on possible increases at earlier ages. Analysis of yearly survey data from the National Survey on Drug Use and Health estimated that the 12-month prevalence of depression in 12-17-year-old youth increased from 8.7% to 13.2% from 2005 to 2017 (Twenge et al., 2019), which may reflect the impact of social media, electronic communication, increasing sleep disruption, and other potential societal changes.

Rates of youth depression have increased substantially worldwide during the COVID-19 pandemic with an estimated one in four youth experiencing clinically significant symptoms of depression (Racine et al., 2021). The American Academy of Pediatrics and the American Academy of Child and Adolescent Psychiatry recently declared children's mental health to be a national emergency (American Academy of Pediatrics, 2021), and the US Surgeon General declared a children's mental health crisis in the US (US Department of Health and Human Services, 2021) with an emphasis on the role of youth mood and depression challenges.

Despite this apparent increase in depressive disorder, there has been no corresponding increase in treatment utilization (Lu, 2019). Along with an overall need for enhancements in the availability of treatment, there are particular disparities for ethnic and racial minority youth in availability of, access to, and uptake of treatment for a range of mental health conditions in youth, including depression (Alegria et al., 2010). There is an urgent public health need for accessible, culturally sensitive, and impactful appropriate interventions for youth struggling with depression to both treat and prevent these disorders.

Depressive disorders *are becoming* *more* prevalent and undertreated, especially for ethnic/racial minority youth

2

Theories and Contributing Factors

Biological and environmental factors contribute to depression

Depression across the lifespan is considered a multifactorial disorder, resulting from the complex interplay of biological and environmental factors. It is heterogeneous with significant individual variation in presentation, symptoms, associated characteristics, history, course, and contributing factors. There are likely many pathways in the development of depression. In this section, we describe some of the major biological and environmental contributing factors, review some prominent models/theories, and then present an integrative model that we have used to help in educating parents about the nature of depression in youth.

2.1. Biological Contributors

Depression includes a range of symptoms and reflects potential dysfunctions in numerous biological systems. While not comprehensive, this section briefly highlights some areas of notable dysfunction, including neural factors, stress response (hypothalamic-pituitary-adrenal [HPA] axis), and genetic factors. Importantly, biological factors, including HPA-axis functioning and neural responses to stress emerge across development and are sculpted by the environment. Parental responses, both negative and positive input, can shape biological response to stressful circumstances, scaffolding the development of neural and endocrine substrates of emotion regulation.

2.1.1 Neural Factors

SSRIs and tricyclic antidepressant medications can improve depressive symptoms in children and adolescents

Monoamines are a group of related neurotransmitter substances, including dopamine, epinephrine, norepinephrine, and serotonin. These substances play a major role in many functions related to self-regulation such as appetite, sleep, homeostasis, memory, and learning. A host of studies have illustrated that disturbances in monoamines may be related to the symptoms of depression and that intervening through medications targeted at changing levels of monoamines has salutary impacts on depressive symptoms. Indeed, there is evidence that serotonin reuptake inhibitors (SSRIs) show benefits for both children and adolescents with depression, and tricyclic antidepressant medications may also have benefits for adolescents with depression

(Cipriani et al., 2016); these studies provide indirect evidence for the role of monoamines in youth depression.

Recent research has focused on understanding the brain bases of depression in adolescents, but few studies have examined preadolescent children. Findings suggest that, relative to youth without depression, youth with depression display smaller hippocampal volumes, decreased cortical thickness of ventral frontal neocortex, reduced functional connectivity between the amygdala and multiple circuits, and increased response to sad faces in parietal cortex (Kerestes et al., 2013). In other words, studies suggest overactivation of brain regions associated with negative emotions and underactivation of brain regions associated with cognitive control (Hankin, 2012). There do not appear to be significant differences between children and adolescents, although the studies are few and samples are small. Interestingly, in addition to youth with depression, these neurobiological differences may also appear in youth at risk for depression as a function of parental depression and may predict onset of depression, suggesting a potential underlying biological risk (Shapero et al., 2019).

Mounting evidence in humans reveals how parental support and criticism may shape their children's brain development, scaffolding the development of these neural substrates related to emotion regulation. A stronger mother-child may promote a more mature neural processing of emotional stimuli (Gee et al., 2014). Alternatively, maternal criticism, a powerful risk factor for depression, is associated with increased activity in brain regions implicated in emotion responding and decreased activity in regions involved in cognitive control and emotion regulation (Lee et al., 2015). Observational studies of parent–child interactions have demonstrated associations between positive or negative parenting and children's brain functions, demonstrating again the powerful interactions between the environment and the developing brain.

2.1.2 Endocrine-Related and HPA Axis

The HPA axis is a crucial biological pathway consisting of the hypothalamus, the pituitary gland, and the adrenal glands. The function of this system prepares us to biologically respond to stressors (fight or flight) by releasing stress hormones (cortisol) that alter the availability of glucose and curb nonessential biological functions. HPA-axis functioning is complex and dysregulation can occur at numerous points in response to stressful events. Measurements of cortisol taken at different points in time can indicate different types of dysregulation. Measures taken at morning wakening are used to assess baseline functioning, and high levels can indicate a chronically heightened stress response system. For measures taken immediately following a stressor or biological challenge, dysregulation at this point can indicate possible over or under response in the face of stress. Measures taken after a challenge can be used to assess the feedback system that allows return to baseline levels after a stressor occurs, and dysregulation at this point can reflect an inability to turn off the stress response. A dysregulated system can result in improper immune system response, inflammation, damage to parts of the brain involved in memory (hippocampus), and other negative impacts.

> Biological factors, such as neural responses to stress, can be shaped by environmental factors

The HPA axis emerges across the course of development and can be powerfully influenced by sleep disturbances, chronic stress, and behavior of caretakers in the environment. Evidence suggests that youth with depression show dysregulations in HPA functioning at numerous points in the stress-response process (Lopez-Duran et al., 2009), and children with currently depressed parents do as well, suggesting that parental depression may impact stress response – a possible pathway through which depression risk may be shaped (Zhang et al., 2018).

2.1.3 Genetic Factors and Parental Depression

Studies of depression in adults suggests high heritability, with the rate for major depressive disorder estimated at about 39% (e.g., Kendler & Prescott, 1999). Compared to relatives of normal controls, relatives of adults with depression show increased rates of lifetime mood disorders. Bipolar disorder tends to run in families of adults with bipolar probands, whereas unipolar depression runs in families of individuals with either bipolar or unipolar depression (Gershon et al., 1982; Merikangas et al., 2014). As detailed below, these findings have been replicated in youth.

Studies of family aggregation of depression have used both top-down or high-risk approaches – selecting depressed parents (mostly mothers) and assessing the risk of mood disorders in their offspring – and bottom-up approaches – selecting depressed youth and assessing the risk of mood disorders in their parents and other family members. The top-down studies indicate that parental depression is associated with risk for both depressive symptoms and disorders in offspring (Goodman et al., 2011); indeed, youth with a history of parental depression, compared to those without a history of parental depression, are about four times as likely to experience a major depressive episode (Avenevoli & Merikangas, 2006). In addition, youth with depressed mothers experience higher rates of diagnosis, recurrence, and chronicity of depression compared to those with nondepressed mothers (Hammen et al., 2012; Weissman et al., 1987; Avenevoli & Merikangas, 2006). Even remitted parental depression seems to increase risk for poorer functioning and more internalizing symptoms (Goodman et al., 2011). Similarly, bottom-up studies consistently indicate that youth with depression have significantly higher rates of depression in their parents as compared to control youth with no mental illness (for review, see Tompson et al., 2015). Findings are less clear when comparisons are made between relatives of youth with depressive disorders and relatives of youth with other psychiatric disorders. Interestingly, studies comparing youth with depressive disorders to psychiatric control groups composed primarily of youth with disruptive behavior disorders (Weller et al., 1994; Kovacs, Devlin et al., 1997; Tompson et al., 2015) were more likely to find significance between group differences in family aggregation of depressive disorders than were studies comparing depressed youth to control groups composed primarily of youth with anxiety disorders (Livingston et al., 1985; Puig-Antich et al., 1989). This could be due to common factors underlying the etiology of youth depression and anxiety.

Genetic studies have identified a number of candidate genes that may underlie vulnerability to depression. The specific genes may impact differences in neural activity, the degree of stress reactivity (e.g., cortisol) in the face of stress, and the likelihood of cognitive biases. A more detailed review can be found in Hankin (2012).

It is important to note that parents contribute both genes and environments to children's development. In examining the association between maternal depression and youth depression, Goodman and Gotlib (1999) describe four potential mechanisms: (1) genetics, (2) neural processes impacting emotion regulation, (3) exposure to negative maternal affect and behaviors, and (4) increased stress in the environmental context. Regardless of the mechanism, from a clinical practice perspective, these data on family aggregation underscore the need to evaluate and consider parents in treating youth for depression. This is particularly true given data indicating a poor response to treatment among depressed youth with currently depressed parents (Garber et al., 2009).

2.2 Child and Developmental Risk Factors

It is useful to consider child and developmental risk factors as both distal and proximal risk factors for depression. Distal risk factors increase risk but may not be related directly to the timing of a depressive episode. These factors increase risk for the emergence of depression over time and include negative early life experiences, social and economic stressors, family functioning, and child temperament and personality. Alternatively, proximal risk factors are best conceptualized as precipitating or triggering events preceding an episode. These factors can vary widely between children and may include losses, specific one-time stressors, and chronic stressful circumstances. To use a gardening metaphor, distal risk factors prepare the soil and proximal risk factors are the seeds of these mental health crises.

Distal and proximal stressors combined can cause cognitive, affective, and social risk factors for onset of depression

2.2.1 Developmental Risk

Early experiences play a significant role in risk for mental health problems in general and can lay a foundation for later emergence of depression. Major stressors for youth-onset depression include early loss of a parent or other significant figure, exposure to poverty and low income, parental incarceration, child maltreatment and/or domestic violence, and parental depression; there is evidence that childhood-onset depression may be associated with greater stress load in early development than adolescent-onset or adult-onset depression (Jaffee et al., 2002). Such stressors are often multifaceted with wide-ranging impacts. For example, parental incarceration may be associated with loss of a parent in daily life and increased risk of low income. As another example, maternal depression may be associated with increased interpersonal stress for both the mother and child.

2.2.2 Temperament/Personality

Temperament describes an individual's biologically based, stable tendencies to react, both emotionally and behaviorally, to environmental events (Rothbart et al., 2000). As an individual develops and the environment shapes these temperamental dispositions, personality emerges. Thus, temperament forms the biological basis of the developing personality. The major temperamental dimensions include negative emotionality, positive emotionality, and effortful control; the corresponding personality dimensions include neuroticism, extraversion, and disinhibition/constraint. According to the tripartite model of anxiety and depression (Clark & Watson, 1991), high negative emotionality/neuroticism is a general risk factor for anxiety and depression, whereas low positive emotionality is a specific risk factor for depression. The combination of temperamental risk – high negative and low positive emotionality (high neuroticism, low extraversion) – places individuals at greater likelihood for the development of depression; this finding has been replicated in studies of children, adolescents, and adults (Klein et al., 2011). It is important to note that despite the impact of early temperamental influence on personality development, events and experiences in the environment have the capacity to impact the developing personality and alter risk for depression (Ormel et al., 2001).

> Development and environmental factors shape temperamental dispositions and can alter the risk for depression

Studies of temperament as a risk factor are complex and point to the challenges of managing emotion in youth. When considering the self-regulatory aspect of temperament by including effortful control along with negative and positive emotionality, we see this complexity emerge. High negativity, low positivity, and low effortful control are each considered risk factors for depression; however, considering them together, being high risk on only one and low risk on any two (e.g., high negative emotionality/high positive emotionality/high effortful control; low negative emotionality/low positive emotionality/high effortful control; low negative emotionality/high positive emotionality/low effortful control), or what has been called the "best two out of three," seemed to be protective. However, in a study of 7–14-year-old youth, the combination of both high negative and high positive emotionality and high effortful control (a possible two out of three) was associated with the greatest increase in depressive symptoms over time (Van Beveren et al., 2019). This combination may indicate that youth with high overall emotionality may engage in overcontrol, in which such youth try to manage, unsuccessfully, these overwhelming emotions. Thus, dimensions of temperament may combine in complex ways to influence depressive symptoms in youth.

2.2.3 Cognitive Contributors

Cognitive approaches to depression emphasize the crucial role of negative thoughts in the etiology and maintenance of depression (Beck & Bredemeier, 2016), including among youth (Abela & Hankin, 2008; Bernaras et al., 2019; Liu & Alloy, 2010). These are based on vulnerability–stress models in which it is proposed that established cognitive vulnerabilities interact with stressful life events or circumstances to result in the development, maintenance, and/or relapse of depressive symptoms or disorders. Cognitive vulnerabilities are negative biases that guide attention, inferences, and memory. A number of cognitive vulnerabilities have been proposed, among them negative cognitive (or inferential) style and negative automatic thoughts. The hopelessness model of depression (Abramson et al., 2013) postulates that individuals hold beliefs that negative events will occur and/or positive events will not occur and that the individual can do little to change this. According to this model, individuals may possess a *negative cognitive style* in which they make internal, global, and stable attributions about the causes, consequences, or self-implications of negative life events. For example, a depressed youth may see failure on an exam as caused by a lack of intelligence – a cause that is unlikely to change (stable), impacts most of their experiences in school (global), and emanates from with the self (internal). Alternatively, a nondepressed youth may attribute this failure to the difficulty of the course – a cause that is situation specific (unstable), is not likely to impact them in other classes (specific), and results from a particular teacher or course material (external). The negative cognitive style renders the individual's perception of the self as incapable of changing the situation – thus a hopelessness model. Beck's cognitive model (Beck & Bredemeier, 2016) emphasizes the role of the "negative cognitive triad" – a set of negative assumptions about the self, the world, and the future – and cognitive distortions in attending to, processing, and remembering information. Individuals possess cognitive schemas that guide attention and memory; the depressed individual has negative cognitive schemas about the world, self, and future (negative cognitive triad) and engages in *negative automatic thoughts and cognitive errors*, including catastrophizing, overgeneralizing, and selectively attending to and personalizing negative aspects of events. Depression in adults and adolescents is associated cross-sectionally with cognitive vulnerabilities, and these vulnerabilities prospectively predict the onset of depressive disorders in the face of negative events (Abramson et al., 2013).

Although studies with teenagers and older children generally provide support for cognitive vulnerability stress models (Turner & Cole, 1994), research with younger children is not always so clear. Cognitive vulnerabilities emerge over the course of development, and children are less likely to have stable cognitive vulnerabilities. Indeed, there is evidence that for younger children negative life events may contribute to the development of cognitive vulnerabilities that later interact with negative events to lead to depression. Put differently, the prepubertal child who experiences numerous negative events

> Depressed youths may attribute the causes of negative events to internal, global, and stable (unchanging) factors

may develop into an adolescent who increasingly attends to, focuses on, remembers, and comes to expect bad things to happen.

2.2.4 Earlier Mental Health Problems

Other mental health problems, like anxiety, can increase the risk for depression

As noted in Section 1.5 on comorbidity, other earlier mental health challenges can increase risk for depression. At the same time this comorbidity can increase risk through genetic or biological pathways, it can also increase risk due to the stresses associated with these other mental health problems. Anxiety disorders, for example, often precede depression, which emerges as the child becomes increasingly hopeless in the face of unresolved anxiety, increasing avoidance, and reduction in pleasurable activities. Indeed, depression is often a result of an unfolding process where the lack of control associated with chronic anxiety eventually leads to a sense of hopelessness and withdrawal. Behavioral disorders, such as ADHD and oppositional defiant disorders, may share genetic risk with depression, and their symptoms can lead to increasing levels of family stress and peer rejection that increase likelihood of depression. Similarly, the stressors associated with academic settings, peers, and family members can contribute to depression in youth with autism spectrum disorders and learning disabilities; in recent years much more attention has been paid to the frequent occurrence of both anxiety and depression in youth on the autism spectrum. Indeed, in explaining the emergence of depression to parents, it is useful to help them recognize how each of these mental health challenges is accompanied by a host of stressors that can lead children to increasing frustration, hopelessness, and isolation that may need to be addressed in therapy for children to show lasting improvement.

2.3 Environmental and Psychosocial Risk Factors

Numerous contextual factors in the environment can increase risk for depression and impact its course. Although not comprehensive, this section focuses on three areas in particular – the stress context, family functioning, and peer relations. These factors are generally not independent. Poor family functioning can increase stress; and stressors like poverty and loss can impact family functioning and peer relationships. Further, this context can impact vulnerability through shaping neural and stress response systems and through influencing cognitive vulnerabilities.

2.3.1 Stress Context

Numerous stressors, acute and chronic, can increase the risk for depression across the life span, including maltreatment, abuse/neglect, exposure to trauma, grief/bereavement/early loss, family conflict and/or domestic violence, low SES, poor academic performance, separation from parents, loss of home/eviction. Compared to adolescent depression, childhood depression is associated with increased childhood adversity, including poverty, stressful life events, parental mental illness, and maltreatment (Shanahan et al., 2011).

Life events can be independent/fateful, in that their occurrence does not depend on the individual's actions (e.g., death of a relative, losing a job due to company closing), or dependent, in that their occurrence is conditioned upon the individual's actions (e.g., ending a relationship, losing a job due to being fired). Depression seems to be particularly associated with a surplus of *dependent rather than independent* life events (Rudolph & Hammen, 1999). Further, these dependent events appear to be *interpersonal* in nature – relationship stressors. Perceived severity and controllability of life stressors have implications with stressors perceived as more severe and less controllable particularly linked to depression (Fassett-Carman, Hankin & Snyder, 2019).

The perceived severity and controllability of stressors can change their impact

2.3.2 Family Functioning

Across childhood and adulthood, risk for, course, and maintenance of depression have strong associations with interpersonal and family processes (Restifo & Bögels, 2009) and are frequently associated with family dysfunction (Tompson et al., 2012), harsh, critical, and angry parental behavior, as well as by low levels of parental support, warmth, and acceptance (Peris & Miklowitz, 2015; Sheeber et al., 1997) – specific targets of our family-based treatment. Notably, these processes predict prospectively such that earlier family processes predict increases in depressive symptoms and onset of depressive disorder (Burkhouse et al., 2012; Lewis et al., 2014; Stice et al., 2004), though some research suggests that the influence between parent–child conflict and depression may be bidirectional (Rudolph & Hammen, 1999). Behavioral genetic research indicates that these associations exist independent of genetic factors (Lewis et al., 2014). A recent simulation study estimated that modifying these parenting practices would reduce onset of youth depression by about 20% overall and 30% in less advantaged families (Lay-Yee et al., 2018).

High parental criticism and anger and low parental support and acceptance predict depressive symptoms

Cognitive vulnerabilities are presumed to be learned responses emerging within family contexts. Interactions with caregivers and others underlie formation of cognitive schemas (representations) of relationships, world, and self. These schemas then direct attention, memory, perceptions, interpretations, and expectations, particularly in interpersonal situations (Baldwin, 1992). Frequent negative interactions/feedback may impede the development of positive schemata and result in negative cognitive schemata – depression vulnerabilities (Cole & Turner, 1993). Garber and Martin (2002) proposed three pathways from parental behaviors to children's cognitive vulnerabilities: modeling, inferential feedback, and general negative, unsupportive interactions. First, through modeling, children may adopt parental cognitive responses to negative events by observing parents' verbal and nonverbal responses. Mothers' and children's cognitive vulnerabilities appear correlated, providing support for modeling as a mechanism. Second, children may develop cognitive vulnerabilities through parents' negative attributions about events in the children's own lives (negative inferential feedback). Alloy et al. (2001) found that, compared to adolescents without a negative cognitive style, those with a negative style reported that parents provided more negative inferential feedback in response to negative events. Among younger children, negative maternal inferential feedback during a laboratory-based task predicted children's negative cognitive style (Mezulis et al., 2006). Third, cognitive vulnerabilities may develop in the context of unsupportive, negative parent–child interactions. High parental criticism and low parental positive feedback and support can lead to a more negative self-concept, reduced feelings of mastery, low expectations for support, and, subsequently, greater depression (Garber & Flynn, 2001).

2.3.3 Peer Stress

Peer stress impacts depression and suicidal ideation, especially for girls and gender and sexual minorities

During late childhood and transitioning to adolescence when relationships outside of the family become an increasingly salient development focus, youth often experience increasing levels of peer stress (Ladd & Troop-Gordon, 2003). Heightened peer stress has been linked with depressive symptoms, particularly for girls (Conley & Rudolph, 2009). Bullying – a severe form of peer stress – may be particularly associated with both depressive symptoms and suicidal ideation both among those who report being victims of bullying by peers and those who report bullying peers (Klomek et al., 2007). With youth increasingly spending time online, cyberbullying has become an additional and significant form of peer stress: Interpersonal aggression that was once primarily confined to school and other peer situations can now reach more fully into the daily lives of youth. Unlike traditional bullying, victims of cyberbullying, but not perpetrators, appear at increased risk for depression (National Institutes of Health, 2010; Kowalski & Limber, 2013). Partly as a function of heightened peer stress, individuals who experience uncertainty about sexual orientation or, especially, gender identity are at risk for both increased depression and suicidality (Guz et al., 2021), particularly in the context of parental rejection and nonsupportive parental responses (Johnson et al., 2020). Although peer stress may increase risk, it also exists with a larger context of child vulnerability and environmental supports. Specifically, girls with executive functioning deficits may be at particular risk in the context of peer stress (Agoston & Rudolph, 2016), as they may lack the skills to manage it. Parental support may buffer the negative impact of peer stress (Hazel et al., 2014).

2.4 Models/Theories

The previously discussed risk factors, both distal and proximal, do not act in isolation. Biological and psychosocial factors influence one another, and environmental stressors may come in bundles. Over the past half century, numerous models have been used to understand depression: Here we highlight three that are particularly relevant for approaching youth depression and influencing our family-focused treatment approach. We then present an integrative model to guide our family intervention.

2.4.1 Vulnerability–Stress Models

Vulnerability-stress models emphasize the existence of vulnerabilities or diatheses within the individual that increase risk for particular forms of pathology (Ingram & Luxton, 2005). In the case of depression, these vulnerabilities may be biological – genetic propensity for dysregulation of neurotransmitter systems (Stockmeier, 2003) – or psychological – negative cognitive style (Abramson et al., 2013). They then interact with environmental stressors to result in the emergence of symptoms. The greater rates of depression during adolescence may be a function of vulnerabilities laid down during childhood interacting with the increases in stress that frequently accompany the adolescent years. Treatments based on this model often include multiple components to treat both the vulnerability, using medications, and the triggering/accompanying psychosocial stressor, using psychotherapy.

Tailored treatments may combine medication and psychotherapy

2.4.2 Cognitive-Behavioral Models

Cognitive models of depression are often conceived of within a vulnerability-stress framework. Negative, maladaptive ways of attending to and processing information about the world, the self, and the future form the vulnerability, and negative events and circumstances provide the stress. Integrating behavioral components, these models emphasize the interplay of thoughts (e.g., negative assumptions, self-statements, causal attributions, hopelessness), behaviors (e.g., social withdrawal, low engagement in pleasurable activities), and emotions (e.g., sadness, lack of pleasure) characteristic of depression. Interventions based on these models emphasize cognitive restructuring to change vulnerability and enhancements in coping to reduce stress.

2.4.3 Interpersonal and Stress-Generation Models

Interpersonal models underscore the crucial role of relationships and the interpersonal context in the development and maintenance of depressive disorders. Indeed, studies suggest that it is not stress in general but rather interpersonal stress in particular that is characteristic and contributory to

Interpersonal models emphasize bidirectionality between interpersonal stressors and depression

depression (Rudolph et al., 2008). A large literature indicates that negative responses and criticism from family members can increase both for emergence and relapse of depression in adults and youth (Peris & Miklowitz, 2015). Stress-generation models posit that the relationship between stress and depression is bidirectional (Hammen, 2006). Depression has a profoundly negative impact on relationships. Depressed youth frequently show significant irritability as well as depressed mood, withdraw from social interactions, blame and criticize others, and repeatedly seek reassurance that goes unheeded. In the stress-generation framework, the symptoms and behaviors of the depressed person contribute to a more stressful, conflictual, and negative interpersonal environment: In turn, the resulting stressors, particularly interpersonal stressors, then fuel symptoms of depression – a classic vicious cycle (Rudolph & Hammen, 1999). Interventions based on this model involve enhancing social and interpersonal skills and coping with and addressing the interpersonal stressors that contribute to symptoms.

2.5 An Integrative Model to Guide Treatment

Figure 1 illustrates a model for thinking about treatment that can be used by therapists conducting psychoeducation with families about mood disorder. The box in the upper left corner emphasizes the role of stressors – peer and family stress and conflict, academic demands, negative life events, medical challenges. The center demonstrates the CBT model – how ways of thinking, feeling, and behaving in response to these stressful circumstances can amplify (and alternatively de-amplify) depressive feelings. Further downward, we see the fueling of symptoms as negative thoughts: Increasingly painful emotions and biological functions become entwined to create a depressive disorder. It should be noted that, although this model has heuristic advantages, the depression does not unfold uniformly in this fashion and can have many other contributing factors as outlined above. Despite its limitations, this model is particularly useful as parents/caregivers consider the types of available treatments that map onto this model, as illustrated in Figure 2.

Interpersonal models can assist in managing the stressors, particularly interpersonal stressors, so frequently associated with depression. CBT models, including problem solving and behavioral activation and cognitive restructuring, can be used to directly address factors that maintain depression. Antidepressant medications can be used to directly intervene in the biological processes underlying depressive syndromes. The model can allow parents and youth to better understand that depression can be addressed through a variety of pathways and that interventions can be combined for maximum benefit.

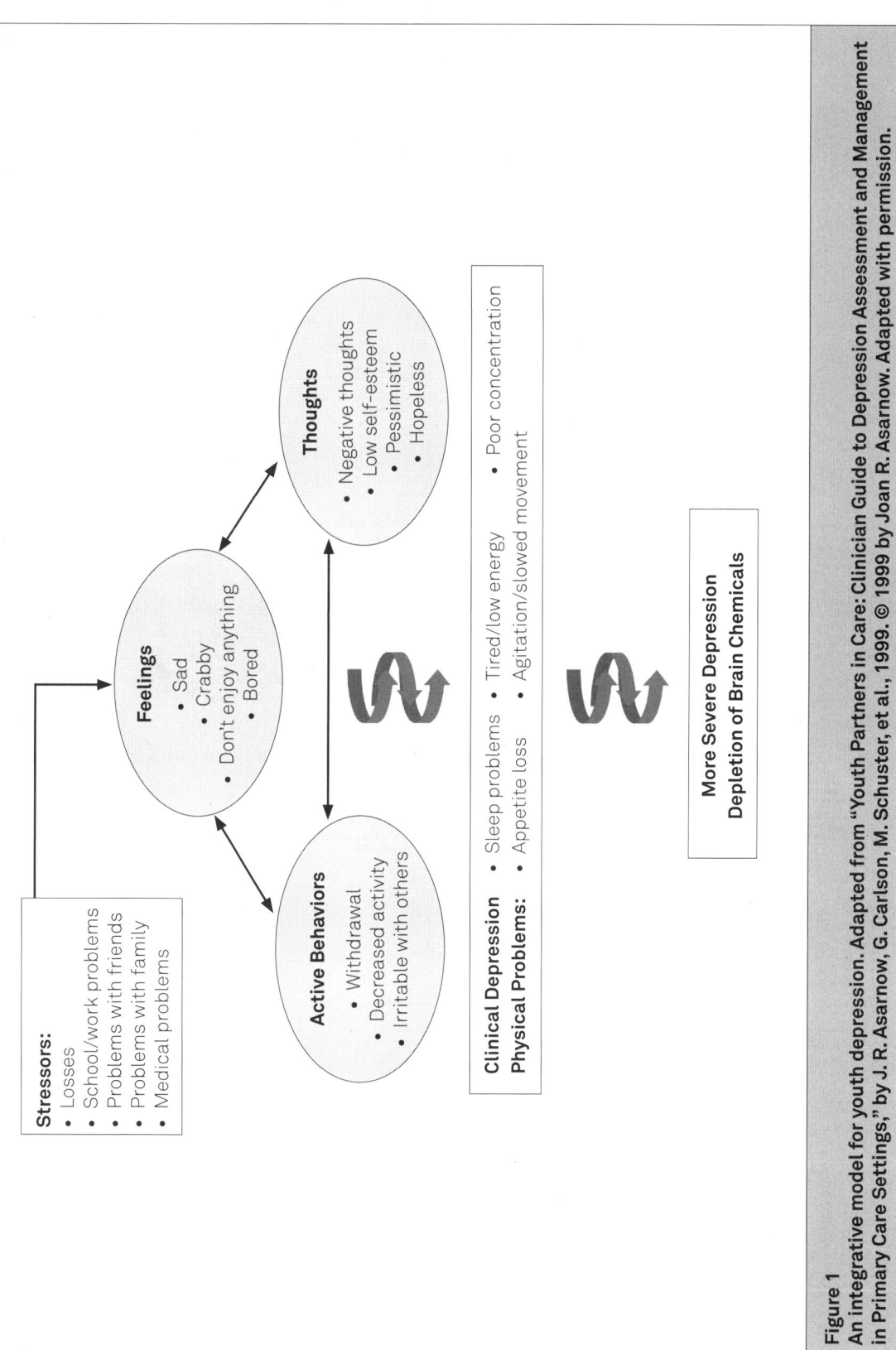

Figure 1
An integrative model for youth depression. Adapted from "Youth Partners in Care: Clinician Guide to Depression Assessment and Management in Primary Care Settings," by J. R. Asarnow, G. Carlson, M. Schuster, et al., 1999. © 1999 by Joan R. Asarnow. Adapted with permission.

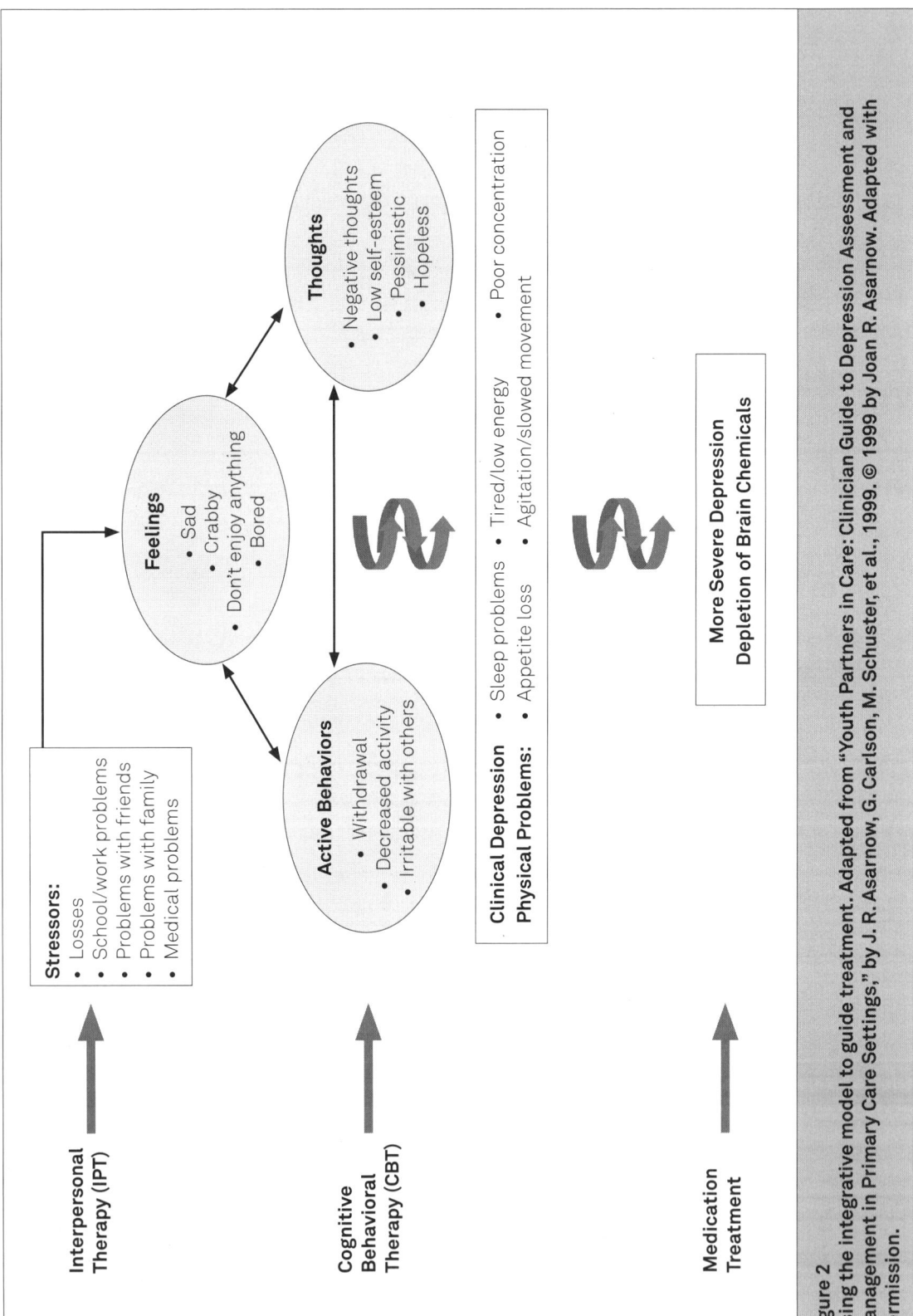

Figure 2
Using the integrative model to guide treatment. Adapted from "Youth Partners in Care: Clinician Guide to Depression Assessment and Management in Primary Care Settings," by J. R. Asarnow, G. Carlson, M. Schuster, et al., 1999. © 1999 by Joan R. Asarnow. Adapted with permission.

3

Evaluation

Evaluation of depression can be conducted using a variety of techniques and should include a variety of reporters where possible. Assessments can include self-, parent-, and teacher-report questionnaires, as well as unstructured, semistructured, and fully structured interviews. As noted previously, depression presents with a range of symptoms, including emotional, behavioral, physiological, and cognitive symptoms; thus, a multi-informant and multimethod approach is recommended to fully evaluate symptoms, their context, and their impact. Combining information from multiple sources can be challenging, and clinicians may have to use their judgment and experience in determining whether particular symptoms meet criteria for a diagnosis of depressive disorders. It should be noted that in addition to clinical information, youth and their family members may have different goals for treatment (e.g., focus on depression or its comorbidities), may prefer different formats (e.g., family versus individual) and may be comfortable with different strategies (e.g., provision of support versus skills enhancement). The American Psychological Association emphasizes the need to consider empirical evidence, clinical expertise, and individual family and patient goals, preferences, and values in implementing a treatment (Langer et al., 2022), and evaluating these family and patient characteristics is necessary.

Multimethod assessment includes child, parent, and teacher perspectives

3.1 Reporters

Parents or other caregivers can supply crucial information on developmental risk factors and emergence of symptoms. Parents/caregivers are in a position to observe the child's behavior at different times of day, on various days of the week, and over long periods of time. Although school personnel and pediatricians may refer youth for treatment, parents/caregivers are most often the source of treatment referral, particularly in prepubertal youth, and their perspective in evaluation and their participation in treatment is essential. Numerous highly reliable and valid assessment techniques have been developed to systematically collect data from parents/caregivers.

Importantly, youth themselves should always be a part of this evaluation. Many symptoms of depression are internal experiences that may not be easily observed by those around the youth. Teenagers in particular are aware of symptoms that parents/caregivers or other adults around them

Youth self-evaluations provide insights into symptoms which may be unknown to caregivers

may not be (e.g., suicidal thoughts) and may be highly accurate reporters on their mood and cognitive symptoms. Children as well provide essential information on their experiences. In addition to providing symptom information, youth provide essential context, including details on peer stress that may be impacting their presentation. There are a number of scales that have been developed to directly assess youth symptoms. It is important to note that older youth may be better reporters of their own symptoms than are younger, preteen children. Few measures have been developed for those under the age of 8 years. In addition, it may be helpful to read the items to younger children, as questionnaires may exceed their reading capacity and, in oral administration, their comprehension of items can be assessed. We have found that including a visual image of the rating scale used can be helpful, giving the child the opportunity to point to the rating that best fits their experience.

Additional provider feedback can give important information in assessing depression. Teachers, guidance personnel, coaches, and others in the academic setting can provide information on current impairment in the school and social environment and speak to stressors that might be contributing to the clinical picture. These informants may be especially useful when comorbidities that impact academic performance are present (e.g., learning disabilities, ADHD). Pediatricians can also be helpful informants, as they may have known the child and family for long periods of time and be able to comment on changes that have emerged across development. Additionally, consultation from a pediatrician can be useful in ruling out potential medical explanations for the symptoms (e.g., thyroid conditions, anemia).

Notably, informants may not always agree on the symptom presentation and associated concerns. Indeed, parents/caregivers who live in the same home with the youth may have different perspectives and concerns. This disagreement alone can be meaningfully related to symptoms, family function, and other important factors (De Los Reyes & Kazdin, 2005). The depression distortion hypothesis posits that depressive symptoms and disorders may alter the perceptions of the individual experiencing the symptoms, influencing their reporting. Depression can impact attention, encoding, and storage processes in memory and thereby influence what is recalled. Given the high likelihood of depressive symptoms and disorders in parents/caregivers of youth with such symptoms and disorders, both reporters may provide information that is colored by their symptoms. Both child and parent perspectives may provide vital information in evaluating mood and functioning in youth with depression (De Los Reyes et al., 2008).

3.2 Special Considerations in Evaluation

Assessment should consider severity, frequency, duration, and interference

Symptoms of depression are frequently more extreme versions of experiences that are widely familiar. Most of us, including youth, have had days, particularly stressful days, where we had little enjoyment in our activities, felt sad and/or discouraged, had little motivation, and experienced doubts about ourselves and our abilities. We may have had times when we had difficulty sleeping due to worries or rumination about negative events and may have lost our appetites as we grappled with a stressful situation. Youth are certainly not immune to these difficult times. Indeed, during pubertal transitions and throughout adolescence as youth grapple with difficult issues of identity formation and relationship development, such changes in mood are not uncommon. Adolescents in particular endorse a wider range of emotional experiences in a given day than do adults (Larson & Sheeber, 2008) and may shift moods more readily. Box 1 lists common warning signs of depression that may be apparent to parents/caregivers, teachers, and others who observe the youth regularly.

Box 1
Frequent Warning Signs of Possible Depression

- Lack of pleasure, interest, enjoyment of activities (anhedonia)
- Increasing irritability (often missed by parents as a symptom of depression)
- Changes in sleep, activity, appetite
- Changes in weight
- Social withdrawal or isolation
- Sadness, crying for no reason
- Vague somatic complaints (e.g., headaches, stomachaches), especially in childhood

---

Given the reality of the frequently increased emotionality of this period of life, when do we diagnose a depressive disorder? Five considerations are particularly important. First, how severe are the symptoms? How bad do they become? Doubts about one's ability and feelings of guilt following a transgression may be common, and potentially appropriate: More severe feelings of worthlessness and self-reproach are characteristic of depression. Second, how frequently do the symptoms occur? Experiencing a night of poor sleep every few weeks, especially when anticipating a stressful event (e.g., test, game, peer interaction) may be common; alternatively, two hours of initial insomnia several nights per week may be more characteristic of depression. Third, how long does it last or what is its duration? Unhappiness or lack of pleasure lasting an hour occurs for many if not most youth, particularly in response to disappointments or setbacks; alternatively, sadness and misery lasting most of the day several days in a row is more characteristic of depression. Fourth, do the symptoms interfere with normal developmental tasks? Occasional lack of motivation and withdrawal may be common; alternatively, avoiding school or peer interactions, decreased academic performance, or disengagement from activities suggest the type of interference and impairment associated with depression. Finally, do the symptoms increase risk? The emergence of self-destructive or suicidal thoughts, plans, and/or behaviors is often indicative of depressive disorder.

Depression and other mental health disorders occur within a cultural, social, and economic context, and APA has emphasized the need to provide evidence-based practice that considers the "context of patient characteristics, culture and preferences" (American Psychological Association, Presidential Task Force on Evidence-Based Practice, 2006). However, there is limited guidance on how to integrate information on culture and context into case conceptualization (Lewis-Fernandez et al., 2020). The Culture Formulation Interview (American Psychiatric Association, 2013) can provide important information to guide clinicians and can help clients to feel that their perspectives are better understood and considered. Sanchez and colleagues (2022) emphasize the importance of considering cultural context and illustrate the use of a five-stage science-informed case conceptualization to (1) assess presenting problems and causal/maintaining contributors and historical factors, (2) diagnose problems, (3) develop hypotheses and a case formulation, (4) select an evidence-based, culturally responsive treatment plan, and (5) continue an individualized assessment of progress.

> A youth's strengths, skills, relationships, and resources are crucial to assess

In addition to evaluating stressors, symptoms, and circumstances associated with depression, clinicians need to attend to strengths, skills, important relationships, and resources in the environment. These factors are often ignored by depressed individuals who, due to increased attention to negative thoughts and circumstances, may not readily report them. Yet, these strengths contribute to an effective treatment plan, providing avenues for intervention. Even the most depressed youth may have areas where they maintain some interests and their functioning is preserved.

3.3 Diagnostic Tools

3.3.1 Depression Screening

> Screening tools are utilized in primary care settings to flag potential mental health concerns

Depression screening tools are frequently used for briefly assessing large populations of individuals for possible signs and symptoms of depression; those who pass this initial screening can then be evaluated in more rigorous ways to assess for presence, severity, and specific symptoms of depression. Screening tools often have high sensitivity (i.e., they pick up most likely cases – true positives) but may have low specificity (i.e., they flag some individuals who do not actually have depression – false negatives). Screening tools are frequently used in primary care or other medical settings as a "first pass." Similarly, brief (5 minute) screenings have been developed on online platforms to flag potential mental health problems (e.g., https://screening.mentalhealthscreening.org/) and can be completed by the youth themselves or parents/caregivers. Table 3 lists and describes common screening tools used with children and adolescents.

Table 3
Selected Screening Tools for Child and Adolescent Depression

Title	Age range	No. of items	Time to complete	Self-report or clinician delivered	Link to measure
Patient Health Questionnaire Adolescent (PHQ-9 A; Kroenke et al., 2001)	11–17	9	5–10 minutes	Self-report or clinician delivered	https://www.med.unc.edu/ihqi/wp-content/uploads/sites/463/2019/03/Adolescent-Depression-Screening-and-Initial-Treatment-Toolkit.pdf
Patient Health Questionnaire-2 (PHQ-2; Kroenke et al., 2003)	11–17	2	Less than 2 minutes	Self-report or clinician delivered	https://www.hiv.uw.edu/page/mental-health-screening/phq-2
HEADS-ED, used in hospital emergency departments (Cappelli et al., 2012)	6–18	7	Less than 5 minutes	Clinician delivered	https://www.psychiatrictimes.com/view/heads-ed-review-mental-health-screening-tool-pediatric-patients
Patient-Reported Outcomes Measurement Information System (Varni et al., 2014)	8–17 Parent report 5–17	8	Less than 5 minutes	Self-report	Introduction to PROMIS: https://www.healthmeasures.net/index.php?option=com_content&view=category&layout=blog&id=147&Itemid=806
Quick Inventory of Depressive Symptomatology Clinician (Rush et al., 2003)	13–17	16	5–7 minutes	Clinician delivered	http://ids-qids.org/

3.3.2 Diagnostic Interviews

The most common way of assessing depression in clinical settings is through an interview. Although a clinical interview can vary widely between practitioners, a number of standardized interviews have been developed to improve diagnostic accuracy by enhancing both reliability and validity. The reliability of an instrument is its ability to yield the same outcome each time it is administered and by each person who administers it. A blood test is reliable if it calculates approximately the same results on two testing occasions close in time; a diagnostic interview is reliable if it yields the same diagnosis in two administrations close in time. By providing a standard set of basic and follow-up questions, a standardized interview improves the reliability of diagnosis. The validity of an instrument is the degree to which it provides an accurate or true evaluation of the phenomenon. A standardized interview may improve validity by providing complete coverage of the symptoms of particular disorders, and strategies for arriving at differential diagnoses. The most frequently used standardized interviews have demonstrated good validity through being compared with other methods for assessing depression. Both reliability and validity are essential in accurate evaluation.

Many of these standardized interviews are conducted with both the parent and youth, as both may provide important information. Youth may be better reporters on certain symptoms (e.g., internal mood states, thoughts) and parents/caregivers may be better reporters of other symptoms (e.g., observable behaviors such as sleep and appetite). Younger children may be less capable of describing their internal states and/or tracking and remembering their behavior, moods, and experiences, and in these cases parental report is crucial. Table 4 lists and describes several common interviews covering depressive disorders in youth.

> **Diagnostic interviews with both youths and parents evaluate symptoms, experiences, and other diagnoses**

These diagnostic interviews have been developed for different purposes (e.g., clinical diagnosis, epidemiological studies) and vary in terms of degree of structure and the role of the clinician in determining whether a response meets clinical criteria. Some interviews are highly structured with all questions asked using specific prompts: Others are more flexible, allowing the interviewer to use a variety of prompts and follow-up questions to assess symptoms. Some interviews rely on the participant to endorse symptoms: Others rely on a trained clinician to determine whether or not a participant's description of symptoms meets clinical criteria. For example, the Schedule for Affective Disorders and Schizophrenia for School Aged Children (KSADS; Kaufman et al., 1997) is a semistructured interview in which the administering clinician is provided with specific questions to ask for assessing specific symptoms of a wide range of disorders in youth – mood, psychosis, anxiety, disruptive problems, elimination, and eating disorders. It begins with an overall screen of core symptoms and, when a youth screens in by providing a positive response, provides additional sections to include more in-depth evaluation of associated symptoms. In evaluating depressive disorders, the core symptoms of depressed mood and anhedonia are included in the screening section: If a youth is positive on these screening questions, the interviewer completes the depressive disorders sections that contain queries for associated symptoms, including questions about severity, frequency, and impairment. The KSADS interviewer needs to have in-depth knowledge of depressive disorders to determine whether the symptoms described meet the clinical criteria. In contrast, the WHO Composite International Diagnostic Interview (Kessler & Üstün, 2004) is fully structured and designed to be administered by lay interviewers.

Table 4
Selected Interviews for Assessment of Youth Depressive Disorders

Title	Age	Subscales	Time to complete	Link
Children's Depression Rating Scale (CDRS; Poznanski & Mokros, 1996)	6–18	None	10–15 minutes	https://www.apa.org/depression-guideline/assessment
Columbia Suicide Severity Rating Scale (C-SSRS; Posner et al., 2011)	Adolescents/teen (10 up)	None	5–30 minutes	https://cssrs.columbia.edu/wp-content/uploads/C-SSRS_Pediatric-SLC_11.14.16.pdf
Diagnostic Interview Schedule for Children-Revised Version (DISC-R; Shaffer et al., 1993)	9–17 years	None	70–120 minutes	https://www.cdc.gov/nchs/data/nhanes/limited_access/interviewer_manual.pdf
Child Interview for Psychiatric Syndromes (ChIPS; Weller et al., 2000)	6–18 years	Child abuse, psychosocial stressors	20–49 minutes	https://www.appi.org/chips-childrens_interview_for_psychiatric_syndromes
Child and Adolescent Psychiatric Assessment (CAPA; Angold & Costello, 2000)	8/9–17 years	Intensity, incapacity, time-related severity	Child mean = 59 minutes Parent mean = 66 minutes	https://psychiatry.duke.edu/research/research-programs-areas/assessment-intervention/developmental-epidemiology-instruments-2
Schedule for Affective Disorders for School-Age Children (K-SADS; Kaufman, Birmaher, Brent, & Rao, 1997)	6–18	None	1–2.5 hours	https://pre.pediatricbipolar.pitt.edu/sites/default/files/assets/AH/AK/KSADS_DSM_5_SCREEN_Final.pdf
Anxiety Disorders Interview Schedule for Children (ADIS-C; Silverman & Albano, 1996)	7–17 years	Unknown	Unknown	https://global.oup.com/academic/product/anxiety-disorders-interview-schedule-adis-iv-child-and-parent-interview-schedules-97801951 86758?cc=us&lang=en&

3.3.3 Depression Symptom Rating Scales

Numerous rating scales have been developed for assessment of depressive symptoms with a list of commonly used ones provided in Table 5. They have the advantage of providing a dimensional rating of depression allowing the assessor to determine severity of symptoms. These rating scales cannot be used to determine diagnosis, but many use a cut score to determine clinical need and provide an estimate of the likelihood of a diagnosable depressive disorder. For example, the frequently used Children's Depression Inventory (Kovacs, 2011) has a range of 0 to 54 and a score of between 17 and 19 is typically considered as the clinical cutoff suggesting a high likelihood of depressive disorder. These scales are often used to evaluate symptoms in individuals at risk for depression, and may be used for secondary screening in a number of contexts (e.g., schools, primary care setting), and are helpful in tracking the impact of treatment.

Table 5
Selected Rating Scales for Child and Adolescent Depression

Title	Age	Time	Reporter	Link
Kutcher Adolescent Depression Scale (LeBlanc et al., 2002)	Teens 12–17	10–30 minutes	Self-report	https://psychology-tools.com/test/kutcher-adolescent-depression-scale
Beck Depression Inventory-2 (Beck et al., 1996)	Teens 13–18	10 minutes	Self-report	https://www.pearsonassessments.com/store/usassessments/en/Store/Professional-Assessments/Personality-&-Biopsychosocial/Beck-Depression-Inventory/p/100000159.html
Center for Epidemiological Studies Depression Scale (CES-D; Radloff, 1977)	Children and teens 6–23	20 minutes	Self-report	https://nida.nih.gov/sites/default/files/Mental_HealthV.pdf
Ohio Scales for Youth (Ogles, 2009)	Youth 12–18 Caregiver 5–18	15 minutes	Self-, parent, evaluator report	https://sites.google.com/site/ohioscales/the-scales
Children's Depression Inventory (CDI-2; Kovacs, 2011)	Children and teens 7–17	5–15 minutes	Self-, parent, teacher report	https://www.pearsonassessments.com/store/usassessments/en/Store/Professional-Assessments/Personality-%26-Biopsychosocial/Children%27s-Depression-Inventory-2/p/100000636.html
EuroQol for Youth (EQ-5D-Y; Devlin & Brooks, 2017)	Children and teens 8–15 Proxy 4–7	5 minutes	Self-report Caregiver Proxy	https://euroqol.org/information-and-support/euroqol-instruments/eq-5d-y-3l/
Mood and Feelings Questionnaire (MFQ; Angold et al., 1995)	Children and teens 6–19	10–20 minutes	Self-report	https://devepi.duhs.duke.edu/measures/the-mood-and-feelings-questionnaire-mfq/

Table 5 Continued				
Title	Age	Time	Reporter	Link
Quick Inventory of Depressive Symptoms (QIDS; Rush et al., 2003)	Teens 13 up	5–7 minutes	Self-report	https://www.braincode.ca/content/quick-inventory-depressive-symptomatology-qids-sr
Depression Anxiety Stress Scales (DASS; Lovibond & Lovibond, 1995)	Teens 14 up	5–30 minutes	Self-report	http://www2.psy.unsw.edu.au/dass/dassfaq.htm
Depression Self-Rating Scale for Children (DSRS; Asarnow & Carlson, 1985; Ivarsson et al., 1994)	Youth 8–14	5–7 minutes	Self-rating	https://www.mcgill.ca/psy/files/psy/depression_self_rating_scale_for_children_dsrsc.pdf
Brief Psychiatric Rating Scale (BPRS-C; Lachar et al., 2001)	3–18	2–5 minutes	Clinician delivered observation items	https://www.smchealth.org/sites/main/files/file-attachments/bprsform.pdf?1497977629
Behavioral Activation for Depression Scale (BADS-SF; Manos et al., 2011)	Young adult; studied in 8–12	10–15 minutes	Self-rating; scored by clinician	https://www.div12.org/wp-content/uploads/2014/11/BADS-SF.pdf
Quick Inventory of Depressive Symptomatology (Self-Report) (QIDS-SR; Rush et al., 2003)	13 to adult	5–7 minutes	Self-report	https://www.mdcalc.com/calc/1845/quick-inventory-depressive-symptomatology-qids
Child Behavior Checklist (CBCL); Youth Self-Report Inventory (Achenbach, 2013)	Children and teens 1.5–18	10–20 minutes	Parent report, self-report	https://store.aseba.org/Child-Behavior-Checklist-6-18/products/19/

3.3.4 Observational and Technological Approaches

Technology provides the opportunity to evaluate signs and symptoms of depression in an ongoing way. Although these approaches are not in typical clinical usage, they show promise. The National Institute of Mental Health (NIMH) Small Business Technology Transfer Program is supporting research evaluating the use of digital monitoring approaches that use smartphones to monitor speech patterns, media usage, activity level, sleep, and other biological indicators that may be useful in management of depression (National Institute of Mental Health, 2020). In one study length of calls, steps taken, and data used were highly associated with depressive symptoms scores among teens with anxiety and depression (Cao et al., 2020). These technology-based approaches may provide an avenue for ongoing assessment of interventions going forward.

3.3.5 Tools for Evaluating Suicidal Thoughts and Behaviors

Evaluating suicidality may be challenging with young children

A number of the previously cited scales include items for suicidal ideation, and the diagnostic interviews include detailed questions. It is always advisable to thoroughly evaluate suicidal ideation in an ongoing way in cases of youth depression. In cases of children under age 10, assessment of suicidal risk is especially challenging, and it is important to assess their understanding of the nature of death (e.g., permanent versus temporary). Table 6 lists important areas of assessment in evaluating suicidal risk in youth, including current diagnoses, symptoms, and circumstances, as well as history. A past history of suicide attempt is the strongest predictor of completed suicide. Fewer measures have been used with younger children. Two in particular bear mentioning. The Child Suicide Risk Assessment (CSRA; Larzelere et al., 2004) was developed specifically for children under the age of 13, includes 20 yes/no questions with some followed up by probes for additional information on endorsed items, and has demonstrated adequate reliability and validity (association with prior attempts). It includes for subscales – worsening depression, lack of support, and death as escape. In general youth had a good understanding of the CSRA items, although there was a steep drop-off from age 7 to age 6, particularly for items assessing comprehension of time and the nature of death. The Child–Adolescent Suicide Potential Index (Pfeffer et al., 2000) was developed for and has been evaluated among both children and adolescents. It has three factors – anxious-impulsive depression, suicidal ideation/acts, family distress – and shows high sensitivity (70%) and specificity (65%). Evaluation and management of suicide risk is an ongoing process in youth with depression.

Table 6
Risk Factors in Evaluating Youth Suicide Risk

Current diagnoses	Current symptoms
Current psychiatric disorder, especially mood, conduct, and/or substance use	Strong feelings of hopelessness and/or worthlessness
Comorbidity of above disorders	Psychotic symptoms
Personality disorder, especially antisocial, borderline, narcissistic	Impulsivity, especially aggressive impulsivity

History	Current circumstances
Previous attempt	Loss of parent or family conflict/discord
Family history of suicide	Availability of lethal means

4 Treatment: A Family-Based Approach

4.1 Evidence Base for Child and Adolescent Depression Treatment

4.1.1 Psychosocial Interventions

Approximately 25 years ago, Chambless and Hollon (1998) proposed a scheme for evaluating the efficacy of psychosocial interventions for mental health problems. Levels of treatment efficacy included well-established, probably efficacious, possibly efficacious, experimental, and questionable. For a treatment to be considered "well-established," it needed to demonstrate superiority to a control group (psychological placebo or active intervention) or equivalent to an established treatment in at least two methodologically rigorous randomized trials by two different investigative teams (Chambless & Hollon, 1998). Both interpersonal therapy (IPT) and cognitive behavioral therapy (CBT) have achieved "well-established" criteria for adolescents (Southam-Gerow & Prinstein, 2014; Weersing et al., 2017). Thus, a substantial literature exists to guide the treatment of depression in adolescents.

There are five levels of treatment efficacy

In contrast, despite evidence of the negative long-term course of childhood depression, the evidence base for preadolescent children is sparser. Recent reviews illustrate the divide in our knowledge of what works for depressed adolescent versus preadolescent youth (Tompson et al., 2012; Weersing et al., 2017). Indeed, in the most recent evidence-base update for youth depression published in the *Journal of Clinical Child & Adolescent Psychology* (Weersing et al., 2017), there were no treatment approaches that surpassed a rating of Level 3: *possibly efficacious* for preadolescent youth, and only a few trials had been conducted. Even among these there were very few with substantial family involvement or focus, although many included periodic parent meetings and brief inclusion of the parent at the conclusion of each session. Thus, family-based interventions for child depression met criteria for only Level 4: *experimental*.

Following the time period covered by the aforementioned review (Weersing et al., 2017), two randomized clinical trials have been published that support the role of family-based treatment for depression in children aged 7–14 years and one for preschool-aged children. Although the specific protocols differ, positive findings from these studies suggest that family-based treatment may now be considered Level 1: *well established*. First, Dietz and colleagues (2015) found that family-based interpersonal psychotherapy (FB-IPT) outperformed child-centered therapy on diagnostic remission and symptom reduction in a sample of preadolescents. FB-IPT focuses on reducing parent–child conflict and interpersonal impairment. Parents/caregivers and children meet with the therapist individually for the first third of treatment and, for the remainder of treatment, sessions are split such that during the second half of each session parents/caregivers, children, and therapists meet together. Second, detailed descriptions of FFT-CD (Tompson et al., 2012; Tompson, Langer et al., 2017; Tompson et al., 2021; Tompson et al., 2020) and reports of its efficacy (Tompson, Sugar et al., 2017; Asarnow et al., 2020) have also been published since. In Section 4.2 we provide a detailed description of the treatment and, in Section 4.4, the efficacy data. FFT-CD differs from FB-IPT in that most of the sessions in FFT-CD are conjoint (parent(s) and child together in the room) with a powerful focus on family interaction. Third, Luby and colleagues adapted the evidence-based parent–child interaction therapy (PCIT) to address the needs of depressed preschool children and their parents (Luby et al., 2012; Lenze et al., 2011). They developed an additional six-session module – emotion development (PCIT-ED) – that specifically targets parental skills to support the child's emotion recognition and regulation and is added to the usual PCIT modules (child-directed interaction and parent-directed interaction). Using a bud-in-the ear microphone, parents are coached to model calm emotion regulation and assist their child in relaxation, labeling behavior and emotions, and navigating intense emotion. Compared to a wait-list control group, PCIT-ED was associated with greater decreased depression severity, reduced impairment, more global improvement, and enhanced emotion regulation over an approximately 6-month period (Luby et al., 2018). These three studies – of FB-IPT, FFT-CD, and PCIT – suggest the utility of family-based approaches to treat depression across childhood and into early adolescence.

4.1.2 Medication Interventions

> Family interventions focus on reducing conflict, providing psychoeducation, and enhancing parenting

As evidenced in a recent meta-analysis (Cipriani et al., 2016), pharmacologic treatments for youth depressive disorders have been evaluated in numerous trials, and SSRIs have demonstrated efficacy for both adolescent and preadolescent youth. In considering antidepressant use, several factors need to be considered. First, practice parameters and guidelines for youth depression suggest the use of an initial trial of psychosocial treatment prior to beginning medication intervention (Birmaher et al., 2007). Second, adolescents and their parents may prefer psychosocial treatment compared to medication treatments for depression (Asarnow et al., 2005), and this preference may be stronger for preadolescents. Third, in 2004 the Federal Drug Administration issued a black box warning for antidepressants as there was some evidence of possible increased suicidal risk associated with SSRIs for those under 18 years old. Despite the small but very real risk of suicide in untreated depressed youth, the issuing of this advisory was followed by a large decrease in prescribing of antidepressant medications (Friedman, 2014). These factors all underscore the need for psychoeducation about antidepressant medications for youth and their parents/caregivers and for effective and acceptable psychosocial interventions for depression. At the same time, several studies support the role of combination treatment for those with significant depressive disorders, particularly those who have demonstrated treatment resistance (see Weersing et al., 2017).

4.2 Family-Focused Treatment for Childhood Depression (FFT-CD)

Our FFT-CD has roots in family psychoeducational approaches, family- and marital-focused treatments for mood disorders developed for adults, and CBT for adolescents. It has also been strongly influenced by interpersonal and stress-generation models of depression (Joiner & Coyne, 1999), which emphasize the bidirectional role of interpersonal stress and functioning as both risk and maintaining factors in depression. The FFT-CD approach views depression in youth as a biopsychosocial phenomenon. Biological and environmental factors contribute to its onset, and negative cognitive processes and interpersonal stress impact course and outcome, leading to a downward spiral of escalating symptoms, negative cognitive processes, and stressful events and interactions. FFT-CD is designed to reverse this downward spiral and provide enhanced support in combating the negative thoughts and feelings associated with depression.

Choosing treatments should involve family psychoeducation and consider child and family preferences

FFT-CD aims to reverse downward spirals of depression symptoms, negative cognitions, and stressful interpersonal interactions

The developmental tasks and context differ between adolescents and preadolescents, and the tasks of the preadolescent years make a family-based treatment particularly appropriate. During adolescence, successful development involves enhanced autonomy from parents/caregivers while simultaneously maintaining a positive parent–adolescent bond, expansion of their social worlds, building skills for independence, establishment of strong and dependable friendships/peer relationships, and managing emerging romantic desires and experiences. In contrast, during middle to late childhood, youth are still strongly dependent on parents/caregivers and other adults to navigate social interactions as they develop social abilities and academic skills. Parents/caregivers provide support and feedback, interface with community institutions on their behalf, and model/teach coping and other key life skills. Children are more strongly embedded in their family environments.

FFT-CD includes CBT and family therapy goals to enhance child's and family coping skills

FFT-CD uses skill enhancement to address and support family relationships. Each of the modules includes both CBT goals – designed to enhance the child's functioning and coping skills – and family therapy (FT) goals – designed to help families develop a more positive view of each member and provide greater, more adaptive support. The specific goals in both the areas are listed at the outset of each module description.

In this chapter we provide potential therapists with verbatim examples (presented in italics) that can be used to introduce and discuss the therapy issues, yet therapists are encouraged to become familiar and comfortable with the approach and use their own words and interpersonal style in implementing the treatment. Reframing family processes and individual behaviors to provide alternative, more positive, interpretations are used often, and the therapist will need to adapt the intervention to the needs of the individual families.

This intervention revolves around skills building for families to improve their functioning and support recovery. Communication enhancement, increasing positive interaction, and improving problem solving are primary areas to be addressed. This therapeutic approach is not a cookbook, but it provides a structure and techniques for addressing issues that families bring into treatment. By providing families with a model for understanding how depressive symptoms may come about and be strengthened, this intervention attempts to help them understand how both negative and positive family interactions can influence mood, how strategies can be developed to change interactions, and how they can improve mood and decrease family stress.

Although this manual includes many specific suggestions for pacing the treatment, the essential point is to attend to the family's particular needs and tailor treatment to these needs. For some families, problems with communication are primary culprits in perpetuating stress, and focusing the majority of effort on communication is appropriate. For some, unresolved problems perpetuate stress, and focusing on these problems is most appropriate. For others, it is the building of more rewarding relationships that is paramount, and fun activities planning may be central. The core of this treatment is on identifying family processes and intervening to improve family functioning. The skills are a means to this end. The treatment is flexible and therapists should not be overly concerned if all the material is not covered with equal emphasis.

4.2.1 Structure of the Therapy

FFT-CD involves primarily parent–child sessions

For all families the process should begin with feedback sessions for both the parents/caregivers and child and one to two family sessions focusing on the core concept of emotional spirals. Although we present the concepts/modules in a default sequence that is typically used, the therapist may adapt the sequence for working with families and children with certain characteristics.

Structure of the Sessions
After the first two meetings, the remainder of the sessions are with the parent(s) and the child. They take on a flexible structure, including each of the following:
- **Meeting with the child.** Each session begins with a brief meeting with the child alone. This provides an opportunity to engage in weekly mood monitoring. A number of techniques can be used to accomplish this. We have often used the Birleson Depression Self-Rating Scale (Ivarsson et al., 1994) covering the prior week. This provides the therapist with an

opportunity to both assess level of depression and monitor suicidality. In addition, the child is able to report issues of concern that arose during the week.
- **Review of week.** Once the parents/caregivers have joined the session, the therapist enquires about the week and notes both highlights and problems that occurred. These are then used later in session when working on skills. This check-in also provides the therapist with an opportunity to model positive feedback skills (Saying What You Liked, Handout 6 in the Appendix).
- **Review of practice.** Reviewing the practice from the previous week provides continuity between the sessions and helps family members to focus on the goals of treatment. All practice review should include family members' subjective reactions to the practice, the degree of success in completing practice, and special attention to problems implementing the practice assignment. If practice was not completed (a common occurrence), it can be done in the session at this point.
- **Presentation of a concept.** The concept that interactional spirals within the family are associated with moods is central to the treatment – the core concept. Each week, examples are introduced of what maintains these patterns and of how they might be changed. The review of the week and practice usually provides material for the implementation of the concept to the family's everyday life. To the degree possible, therapists should use material from the family to discuss concepts. The question is, "How does the model help us understand what is happening in this particular family?"
- **Implementation of new concepts.** This occurs each session through the use of role-plays, problem-solving exercises, and discussion. Role-plays give family members a chance to practice skills and "try on new hats." Therapist modeling helps members learn the new behaviors and also puts them at ease prior to the role-play. Let's Play It Out is a role-play game frequently used to work on new communication skills. Family members draw cards from a bag. Each card has a statement written on it, and family members are to practice the skill on an issue raised on the card. Some examples are included in Appendix 3, but additional practice opportunities and prompts can be developed depending on the family need and developmental needs of the child. Discussion of how the concept might operate within the family helps members understand the relevance of the material to their particular situation and apply the concept. Problem-solving exercises allow family members to solve specific family problems and practice new skills in negotiation and problem resolution.
- **Practice assignment.** The goal of practice assignments is to encourage generalization of communications and problem-solving skills to home life.

> Families conduct role plays, problem-solving exercises, and discussion to understand and model new skills

Number of Sessions
FFT-CD is a flexible intervention that can be implemented in approximately twelve 75-minute sessions or fifteen 50–60 minute sessions. As outlined in Table 7, the number of sessions devoted to each of the five modules (described

Table 7
Sample 15-Week Format

Module	Session	Session content
Module 1: One Way to Understand Depression	1	Meeting with parents
	2	Meeting with child
	3	First family session: interpersonal model
Module 2: Families Talking Together	4	Positive feedback
	5	Active listening
	6	Negative feedback
	7	Practice of communication skills
Module 3: Things We Do Affect How We Feel	8	Identifying pleasurable activities
	9	Asking for what you want
Module 4: We Can Solve Problems Together	10	Identifying problems
	11	Taking emotional temperature
	12	Problem-solving model
	13	Practice of problem-solving skills
Module 5: Saying Goodbye	14	Review of progress
	15	Problem solving for maintaining change

The family members participating in each session can vary over time

in Section 4.2.4) will differ depending on overall treatment length. Both formats have been implemented effectively with families in our work. Table 8 illustrates a sample 15-week format to illustrate how session content might be managed in this format. Throughout treatment there may be times when an individual session with the parents/caregivers or child is warranted. Families should be made aware of this from the beginning and such sessions should be normalized, for example:

Although we'll all meet together most of the time, sometimes it's good to have a session with just [child's name], like at the beginning, when I meet with each of you separately. Most families find this helpful, but your family is unique, so we'll have to see what will be most helpful to you.

The therapist will then have more flexibility to address family issues as they arise.

Table 8
Session Content for 12- and 15-Week Treatment Formats

Module	12-week format, no. of sessions	15-week format, no. of sessions
Module 1: One Way to Understand Depression	3	3
Module 2: Families Talking Together	2–3	3–4
Module 3: Things We Do Affect How We Feel	1–2	2–3
Module 4: We Can Solve Problems Together	3–4	4–5
Module 5: Saying Goodbye	1–2	2

4.2.2 Important Treatment Strategies

The following is a list of some of the most important treatment strategies:

- **Exploring antecedents and consequences.** By identifying downward and upward spirals, families begin to understand the antecedents and consequences of problem behaviors (depression, acting out). This enables the family to more clearly see the interactional nature of depression, to identify high-risk situations, and to develop preventive strategies.
- **Personalize information.** Communication and problem-solving exercises must address relevant and important family issues, as this helps the family recognize the utility of learning the new skills.
- **Frequent reframing.** Reframing gives family members a new, more positive interpretation for behavior in the family, allows members to feel less stressed and guilty, and emphasizes family and individual strengths.
- **Normalizing.** By emphasizing that the family's difficulties and challenges are normal and expected, this strategy reduces stigma and helps family members to trust the therapist as someone who will not judge or blame.
- **Removing the child from the identified patient role.** This intervention identifies family interactional patterns as the focus and provides a rationale for the structure of the treatment. This is accomplished by (a) reframing the problem as a family issue and (b) asking the child's feedback on role-plays and in problem solving so that the child can try out a new family role as a member with something to contribute rather than the one with the problem.
- **Involving disengaged members.** When beginning role-plays and discussions, it is important to involve more distant and disengaged members, thus increasing their interactions with other family members. Therefore, if two members have little interaction with one another, the therapist tries

to increase their level of positive contact, either in session (role-plays) or out of session (practice assignments together).

- **Supporting differentiation and family hierarchy.** While encouraging families to work together, it is also important to be supportive of appropriate autonomy between the members. Children (especially those approaching, entering, or navigating puberty, or postpuberty) may need and want to solve problems on their own, and parents/caregivers may have problems that need to be solved within the parental subsystem alone. These boundaries need to be respected and encouraged. This issue may often be addressed in problem solving, where it will be important to identify issues that are appropriate and/or inappropriate for problem solving within the family context. At times, an individual session with the child may be important (e.g., to work on problem solving around a specific peer problem) and a joint session with parents/caregivers may be essential (e.g., when marital or parenting problems interfere with treatment implementation or are clear family stressors). Box 2 gives examples of where individual sessions are particularly appropriate.

Individual sessions with parents and children allow feedback at the appropriate developmental level

---

Box 2
Indications for Scheduling Individual Sessions

Individual parent session

- Serious conflicts over parenting/discipline or need for specific child management techniques
- Marital conflict inhibiting effective intervention or parents considering marital separation
- Parents need education (e.g., normal child development) to establish appropriate expectations
- Suicidality or other safety concerns

4.2.3 Setting the Stage with Individual Sessions

The first two sessions set the stage for the family-based intervention. The clinician should meet individually with the parents/caregivers and with the child. These sessions are presented to the family members as an opportunity to provide feedback about the evaluation. Issues to be addressed with both parent and child include (1) feedback on the evaluation, (2) confidentiality (and how this will be handled within the family), (3) the rationale and goals of treatment, and (4) any additional individual/family concerns that impact the situation. As the level of dialogue and need for specific types of feedback may vary significantly for parents/caregivers and children, these interventions ideally are conducted in two sessions conducted sequentially on the same day – one with the parents/caregivers and one with the child.

Session 1: Meeting With Parent(s)

> **CBT goal:** Provide psychoeducation about depression to support the role of parents/caregivers as models for their children and help them feel empowered to help their child.
>
> **FT goal:** Emphasize the role of "stress" in perpetuating family difficulties and child symptoms, refocus from "fixing" the child to helping the family to cope with stress.

Giving Feedback About the Evaluation

This session begins by providing the parents/caregivers with feedback on the evaluation, including diagnoses, a brief conceptualization of the case (emphasizing the role of stress), and treatment recommendations. Although each conceptualization will differ depending on life circumstances, comorbidity, and other factors, each needs to include a description of the current symptoms, a review of some of the stressors that might be contributing to the symptoms, and a model for how the symptoms came about (again emphasizing stress, which the whole family is experiencing). This example here integrates these pieces:

In reviewing all the material about [child's name] it sounds like a lot has been going on in the last few months (years ...). There are many difficulties both you and [name] have been dealing with and he/she/they has/have been experiencing some symptoms of depression. When kids get stressed, they sometimes have these symptoms – things like having trouble sleeping, feeling really down and grouchy, believing things just aren't going to get better, and feeling like they are not good people [any relevant symptoms]. It seems like after [child's name] grandmother died, the whole family went through a hard time [description of events] ... [child's name] started feeling pretty bad, he/she stopped doing the fun things he/she enjoyed and things just got worse. Does this sound like what was happening?

For families who would like more information on the nature of depression the Symptoms of Depression and the How People Get Symptoms of Depression handouts (Appendix 2) may be used.

It is particularly important to understand the parents/caregivers' perspective on the child's difficulties. Parents/caregivers may not view the child's depression as the foremost difficulty: This is particularly important in cases of diagnostic comorbidity. Indeed, with a child experiencing disruptive behavior problems as well as depression, the irritability and difficult behavior may be foremost in the minds of parents/caregivers. In this case it is important to help the parent see the relationship between the behavioral problems and the child's feelings and to reassure them that the therapy will address the behavior as well.

With parents only, the therapist provides feedback and presents the treatment rationale and goals

Rationale for Treatment

During feedback, the parents/caregivers need a rationale for why this treatment is important and useful. First, we emphasize the important role that the parents/caregivers can play in helping the child learn to cope more effectively. We stress that this is a teaching situation, as shown in the following:

Parents often feel helpless when their kids get down and are having some trouble. As strange as it may sound, we think parents can be pretty powerful. Parents are the most important people in their children's lives, but sometimes they just don't know what to do. Parents have often tried many things and feel like nothing is working. As parents, there are some things you can control and some things you can't. It may not always be possible to help [child's name] when he/she's going through a hard time, but lots of times there are ways to help. In this treatment we work with kids and parents who are going through stressful times to try out some new strategies for coping. When one person in a family feels stressed, it is hard on everyone! So we feel it is important to work together. Sometimes parents tell us they don't know what to do, that they are out of ideas. Do you ever feel this way? You learned certain ways to deal with your stress that have worked for you, and as parents you have helped your kid to learn how to cope with stress. We're going to work on helping your family become even stronger and find extra ways of coping during these hard times. Part of your job here will be to help you and your child learn new ways to cope.

Predicting difficulty helps prepare parents for the inevitable problems associated with the treatment process. The therapist can return to this in later sessions when difficulties arise, for example:

It's never easy to try to make changes. It may be hard to try out new strategies. It can be particularly tough when you are feeling frustrated. We're also learning from one another. Your family is unique. Some things we do may work for your family, but others may not work as well. You'll have to really be honest about letting me know what is working and not working for your family.

Second, demonstrate the thoughts, feelings, actions model (Handout 1). Emphasize that stress can cause many kinds of changes – affectively, cognitively, and behaviorally:

When kids are experiencing stress, they sometimes get to feeling down or irritable, they think badly about themselves, and they start to act differently. This model can help us understand how it works. So you see, stress can affect your feelings and actions and thoughts, which then influence each other. For example, kids start to feel down about things (feelings), then they may blame themselves (thoughts), and they may then start avoiding other kids (actions). This often only makes them feel worse. It's like getting into a big rut. You can really start anywhere and it keeps going around. For example, if a kid feels down and depressed (feelings), he sometimes stops doing fun things (actions), then he thinks "nothing good ever happens to me" (thoughts) and he feels even worse. Can you think of a time you've seen something like this happen with [child's name]?

> It is important to build parent's understanding of their role in the treatment

Third, we want to facilitate the development of greater empathy for the child. This empathy can be used to help parents/caregivers connect with their child and to the treatment process, particularly for parents/caregivers who themselves have experienced depression. An example would be:

Actually, this happens to adults as well as kids. Can you think of times when stress got to you like this? What do you do to deal with stress? Have you ever had the kinds of feelings [child's name] is experiencing? What have you done to try to cope with it? What happened then? Do you know anyone else who has had this happen to them? You can use these experiences and what you know about them to help your kid.

Finally, we want to emphasize strengths and get away from a pathology model:

When kids are going through stress they can have a hard time, but they usually have things going for them that help. What are [child's name] strengths? What does he do well? What is she good at?

The therapist may help parents/caregivers see strengths if they have difficulty. The therapist may reframe the child's negative behavior to emphasize its potential upside. For example, for a child who is "stubborn" the therapist may reframe as:

Your son is someone who can really stand up for what he thinks is right: It sounds like in the future this could help him really stand up for what he knows is right. These are things we can really use to help out in working as a family.

Housekeeping and Setting Up the Frame

The schedule for sessions should be laid out. The issue of confidentiality will need to be addressed, and parents/caregivers should be informed that while it is important to keep the child's confidentiality after the initial individual sessions, any information of concern would certainly be brought to their attention. An agreement about confidentiality should be reached prior to the session with the child. Finally, the parents/caregivers should be reminded that after each session there will be practice: The importance of this practice for the progression of treatment should be emphasized.

Session 2: Meeting With Child Alone

> **CBT goal:** Provide a model for understanding how good and bad feelings are related to thoughts and behaviors.
> **FT goal:** Prepare the child to meet with the parents/caregivers in a constructive, problem-solving situation. Take the focus off the child as the problem and refocus it on working as a family to fight depression.

Transitioning From the Evaluation

Depending on the age of the child, this evaluation may involve more play or focus on discussion. Establishing initial rapport, providing a rationale in the child's language, incorporating their goals and viewpoint, and instilling hope are the goals. The meeting often begins by asking how the evaluation was experienced by the child:

You've sure had to answer a lot of questions in the last couple of weeks when you came here. Some kids like it, but other kids don't. What did you think of all these questions?

If the child was upset, irritated, or had other negative feelings this should be addressed:

It sounds like this wasn't much fun for you and made you feel [name feeling]. I'm sorry it was so tough, but I really want to thank you for being so patient. You did a great job. It's over now and we're going to be having some meetings with you and with your parents together without all those questions. What do you think of that?

If the child expresses negative feelings about the sessions, reassure them that they will not be the focus of blame:

I can see why you might not want to come, especially if you get blamed for stuff. We don't think kids are to blame at all for problems. What we really want is to help you and your parents find ways to make things go easier at home so that everyone is happier. I hope you will give it a try.

The therapist can then normalize the child's feelings of sadness and/or anger, providing a setting where the child is less likely to feel stigmatized. Using the child's words/language helps the child feel understood. The child may have their own labels for the emotions they feel.

Building a Model for Understanding Stress and Pain

> Visuals – notepads, colored pencils – are used to model the child's understanding of emotions and stress

The therapist should be working with the child to understand their point of view, letting the child know that you want to hear about their experience, making them a collaborator in the treatment process, and conveying a strategy for removing the pain. These processes are central to this part of the second session. The child needs to feel understood. The following is an example of a potential conversation:

You told [or your parents told] [evaluator's name] that there is a lot of stress right now. Some people think that kids' lives are really easy and fun all the time, but we think life for kids can be stressful and hard sometimes. Kids have problems too, just like grown-ups! When kids have a lot of stress they have all kinds of thoughts and feelings. But you are your own kid, and I'd like to understand what things help you feel good and what stresses you out.

A beginning focus on the positive will help (1) assure the child that treatment will not focus exclusively on negative things and (2) help them recognize the positive feelings of which they are capable. Taking an emotional temperature gives a sense of how powerful the feelings are. Writing the model on a large notepad or, when possible, having the child do so, can help focus the activity and involve the child.

To specify both sad and happy times, we first show children a group of colored pencils and ask them to pick out the one that seems like the happiest color, one that seems like the saddest, and one that seems like the maddest color. We discuss what makes the color seem to evoke that feeling. We then ask them to remember a specific time they felt like that color. We then discuss each feeling and example in turn using the thoughts, feelings, action model (Handout 1). A potential conversation could be:

Can you remember a time you felt really good and happy, like this color? From 1 to 10, how good were you feeling? It sounds like some good things were happening. When kids are going through good times they have all kinds of feelings. What were you feeling? I'm going to write it down on this paper. When kids are feeling good they do all different things, some jump up and down, some tell their parents all about it, some just smile a lot. What do you do when you are feeling really good? When kids are feeling really good they have all kinds of thoughts. Sometimes they think "life is great," sometimes they think "I'm a great kid." What kinds of thoughts do you have when you are feeling good?

Can you remember a time when you felt really bad, like the color of this pencil? When kids are stressed out they have all kinds of feelings, some kids feel sad, some feel mad, and some feel lots of other things. How do you feel when you are stressed out? I'm going to write this down on the paper. When kids have these feelings they do different things. Some kids I know stop spending time with their friends, others just go to their rooms, and others fight with their parents or brothers and sisters [use relevant examples]. What do you do? When kids have these "stressed out" feelings, they can also have all kinds of thoughts. Some kids think "things will never get better," some kids think "I'm just bad." What do you think about when you are stressed?

The goal here is to help the child to build a model for understanding stress and pain and explain how the treatment is going to help these things go away. Helping the child summarize this process from their own perspective is the goal here:

So it sounds like when the kids at school are mean to you, you feel very sad, go home and stay in your room, and just think "nobody is ever going to like me." Well, we're going to work with your parents so this doesn't happen so much. We might not be able to make things perfect, but I sure think we can make things better. What do you think?

The child may express hopelessness at this point, and this should be addressed with encouragement:

It sounds like sometimes it feels hopeless, like it will never get better. When kids are stressed out sometimes it's hard to see things getting better. But if we all work together maybe we can find some new ways.

Finally, before the session ends, the child will need to be informed of the limits of confidentiality, and their concerns in this regard should be explored. Where children clearly do not perceive a link between family and other interactions and mood, it is appropriate for the clinician to implement mood monitoring practice (Mood Monitoring, see Appendix 2) to assist the child in linking mood to ongoing life events/circumstances. This may be included as homework.

With the child, the therapist focuses on building hope, validating feelings, and shifting away from blame

4.2.4 Family Sessions

Each of these sessions should involve the parents and child. We have sometimes also included siblings for some or, in a few cases, all sessions. When there is a preschool sibling, having them attend sessions increases the likelihood that both parents/caregivers, where available, can attend as well. By including some toys in the room, we have found that it is not too difficult to manage the younger sibling. With older siblings including them can be particularly useful to manage sibling conflicts and build broader skills. The decision about how many sessions may need to include siblings is made on a case-to-case basis, considering economic realities (e.g., no childcare) and the conceptualization of the individual family.

Module 1: One Way to Understand Depression

> **CBT goal:** Present model for understanding depression and rationale for family approach to treatment.
>
> **FT goal:** Remove child from identified patient role. Establish the family as the unit of treatment by reframing the problem as an interactional one.

Introduction to FFT-CD Using the Core Concept: Emotional Spirals

In this session the shift is strongly toward an interpersonal framework, emphasizing that feelings and interpersonal behavior go together. Handout 2 (in the Appendix) is useful to present at this point. The session can begin:

I want to thank you all again for coming here today. Being here together really tells me how much you care about each other. The first thing I wanted to talk about today is one of the ways that people get to feeling down and then get more and more depressed and feeling bad. Once we understand how it happens, we can all do things to keep it from happening, so that everybody feels happier. How does that sound?

As strange as it may sound, the way we feel and the way we do things sort of go together. See this? Feeling bad can start here at our own feelings, at how we act toward others here or how others act toward us here. Sometimes it's hard to change the feeling part, you know by just trying to feel better. It's easier to change the things we say and do when we're with one another.

Now the discussion can move directly to the Downward Spirals diagram (Handout 3). A sample downward spiral is included in Figure 3. The conversation could be:

See, it goes like this: You're feeling bad, so you're not nice to someone; then they are mean back to you and you feel worse. This is a downward spiral, and it just keeps on going. See how it works? This happens in every family. Can you think of a time it happened in your family?

At this point an innocuous therapist self-disclosure can be useful to normalize and make it more concrete. The Figure 3 example can also provide a good discussion. Use the family's example to discuss what happened and how it made each person feel. Ask each family member to give an example but be careful not to let members nag one another. This should be brief, light. Reframe intentions as good and emphasize each person's real and understandable frustrations. Moving on to the positive is important here. Problems will be addressed more in detail throughout the treatment, but this session should really emphasize the positive. Now the focus can move directly to upward spirals using Handout 4:

The good news is we can also get these spirals to go up. Like when you feel happy and do something nice for someone and then they give you a hug, and you feel even

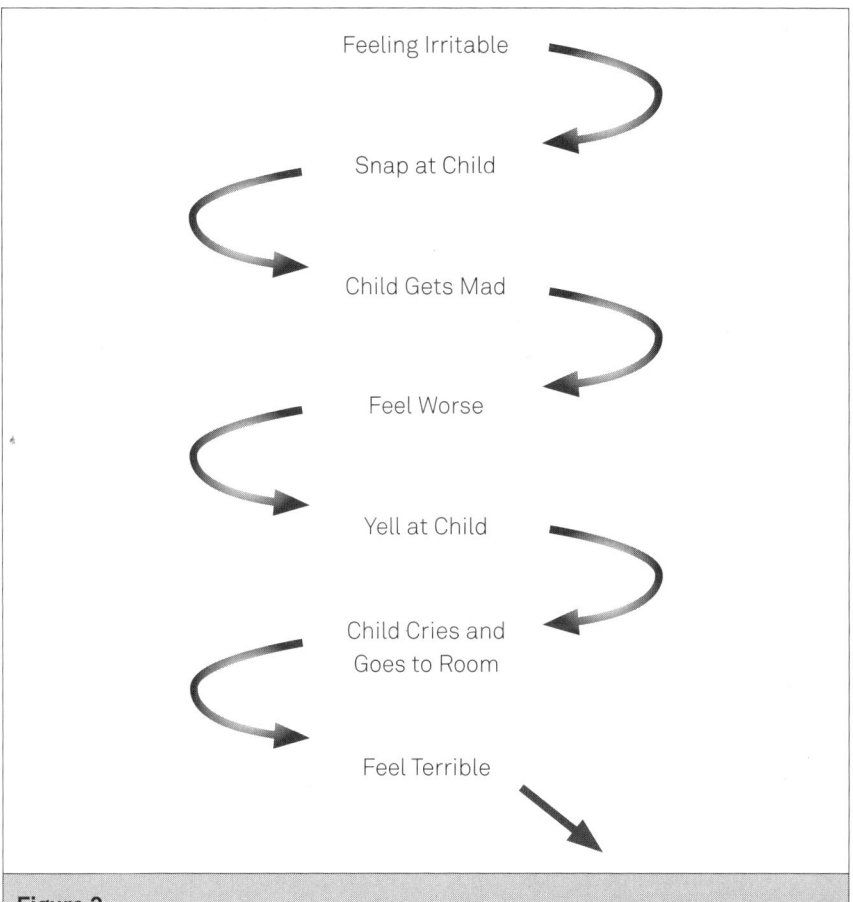

Figure 3
Sample downward spiral. A blank version is available in Handout 3.

better. See this picture? At this point in the spiral you feel pretty good. Can you think of a time this happened in your family?

Figure 4 provides an example of an upward spiral. As with downward spirals, ask each family member to give an example. Discuss what happened and how each person felt about it. Sometimes family members have trouble coming up with upward spirals. Normalize this – when families have been under stress sometimes they get overly focused on problems and forget to notice the positives. Even small upward spirals can be a jumping off point; sometimes upward spirals with pets can be a good avenue as well. Throughout the treatment, the therapist needs to be aware of family interaction patterns that influence the specific spirals and be ready to tailor the intervention accordingly. For example, when one parent is only peripherally involved in daily family life and conflict between the child and other parent brings the family together, the therapist may point out the pattern, talk with family about the pros and cons of that strategy, and problem solve new ways for coming together as a family.

When it is hard to identify upward spirals, small moments (e.g., a hug, playing with pets) can be a good start

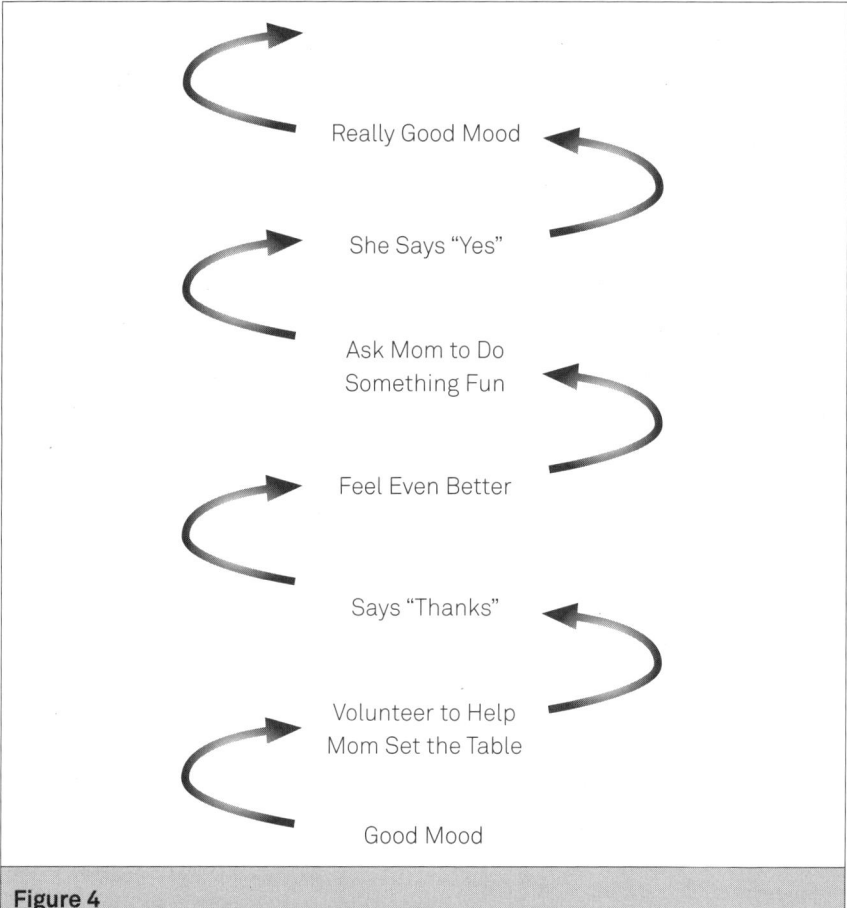

Figure 4
Sample upward spiral. A blank version is available in Handout 4.

Specify the Treatment Goals

This is the core concept, the rationale guiding all treatment – *to stop downward spirals, to start upward spirals, and keep them going.* We have found this treatment rationale to be one that parents and children, even young ones, can relate to. All the interventions then come back to this core idea – we learn skills to help manage these upward and downward spirals:

When kids and parents feel upset sometimes, the way they talk to each other, the way they feel about each other, the things they do together, and the way they solve their problems together, these things can make things turn into an upward spiral or make things go in a downward spiral.

The reason for and the focus of today's session is how family members can help each other to turn downward spirals into upward spirals, namely letting someone know when you like something they do, they say, or just something about them.

One of the primary goals of therapy is to help family members be better observers of their own interactions, and sessions provide a useful opportunity to work on this observational process. The therapist can help family members to identify downward spirals, label them, and use them as training exercises.

> Goals are to identify upward and downward spirals, increase positives, and reduce blame

For example, the therapist may observe and describe a downward spiral and, in an empathic way, the therapist can then help the family chart the spiral and think of new ways to stop it. Active intervention on the part of the therapist can reduce scapegoating in session and help families focus on their interactions.

Giving Positive Feedback During the Sessions

This is a critical skill that family members are learning and should be modeled throughout. We have adapted (modeled on Rotheram-Borus et al., 1994) the use of tokens in the intervention. The tokens here are a form of communication rather than as a way of earning points or credits. The idea of the tokens is to let others know that they did something that you liked and for families to begin to increasingly notice and acknowledge positive family member behavior. Rather than try to collect or earn tokens (and in contrast to typical token economy approaches), family members are encouraged to given them all away. Brightly colored poker chips are typically used as tokens:

One of the things we do in this treatment is that we all get tokens whenever we do a good job, like when you come up with a really good idea. So I'm going to give everyone five tokens, and when someone says or does something you like, give them one. This is how we reward others for doing a good job. OK?

We've practiced some. Now what does your family do to help when you are in a downward spiral (or what would you like them to do) that turns it into an upward spiral?

Ask each family to list at least two things for each other family member. The therapist should help the child at this point, particularly with writing the ideas down.

While chips work well with school-aged children (8–10 years), they sometimes work less well with older preadolescents and young adolescents. For these youth it is important to use humor and modeling: With this approach most older preadolescents can enjoy this exercise. We have also found that we can use brightly colored sticky notes on which family members can write a brief message – thanks notes. These thanks notes can be used in the course of daily life – on a lunch box, a pillow, a bathroom mirror – as well as during sessions. Many of our older youth prefer this strategy. It can also be useful to complete a problem-solving exercise in which the family works on ways to let others know, either verbally or nonverbally, what they have done that is liked or appreciated. With particularly nonverbal kids, this nonverbal solution (tokens) may provide an initial means to initiate more active communication training. The goal of this exercise is to create more positive communication.

Exchanging colorful poker chips and sticky notes can help recognize positives and show appreciation

Practice: Catching Upward Spirals

At the end of this session we send each family member home with five tokens with the goal of giving them all away. Sometimes family members will ask what to do with the ones they get from others: Instructions are to keep giving them away. This then becomes a game that family members can engage in throughout the week to catch and reward upward spirals. This game can become one that family enjoy, and we have found that it invokes some laughter, as the tokens are found under the seat of the car or other unexpected places, leading to intensification of this game. We ask each of them to complete an exercise in which they document the upward spirals throughout the week – Catching Upward Spirals (Handout 5 in the Appendix). Sometimes family members will state that they do not have these in their family: We insist that the goal here is to start noticing the little things that others do in the family – the spirals happen, we often simply fail to notice the positives around us. We explain this in the following way:

Every week I'm going to assign you all just a little practice. It's not hard, it doesn't take much time, and it can be fun. Your practice this week is to try really hard to notice when someone in the family starts an upward spiral. They could start one just by being nice, by helping out, or by smiling.

Here's a log, everyone try to write down something every day that started an upward spiral. Where is the best place in your house to keep this log so that everyone can remember to write something down. Also, I'm going to give everyone five tokens. When someone does something nice this week, give them a token. The goal is to give all your tokens away by the next time we meet. Thanks again for coming this week!

Module 2: Families Talking Together

This module is two to three sessions.

> **CBT goal:** Increase child's assertiveness skills and decreasing depressive withdrawal and irritability.
>
> **FT goal:** Engage family members and encourage the development of empathy between members.

Review of Homework

Each session starts with a review of positive family events/interactions

Always review practice. If they did their practice, praise family members for their efforts – this provides an opportunity to model the Saying What You Liked skill (Handout 6 in the Appendix) – and use the tokens for each family member. If they did not do their practice, have them do it in the session, but reframe their resistance, for example:

It sounds like you were all really busy this week. Keeping track of the good things can be a real effort for all families. Let's think back over what happened this week and try to write down at least two things that each person did that we liked.

For many families spending a few minutes at the beginning reviewing the positive events of the past week starts the session off nicely, so we begin each session this way. These sessions are focused on communication training and are best done with significant role-playing. We have included specific suggestions and cautions for role-playing in Table 9.

Communication Training: Positive Feedback

Use the upward spiral idea to present the rationale for working on positive feedback. Although the example below has the therapist going over each

Table 9
Role-Play Suggestions and Cautions

Suggestions	Examples
Set the scene – use real life examples.	*Let's pretend that Marie just got home from school ...*
Role-play the statement.	*Say it just as if that were happening now. What would you say?*
Getting feedback from other family members.	*What did Angela do well? Where could she make it better?*
Model the statement for the family.	*So it might sound like this ...*
Rehearsal – have family members try again.	*Let's try again, adding how it would make you feel.*
Coaching – suggestions for improvements.	*It would be helpful to be more specific.*
Reinforcement – praise attempts.	*Good job saying how it would make you feel!*

Cautions	Examples
Don't force anyone to role-play, move to another person in the family or model it.	*Let's start with Mom then? Maybe I can demonstrate how you might say it.*
Role-playing can be awkward, remind that it is a good way to learn new skills.	*This can feel a little weird sometimes, but it helps us learn to do it better.*
Don't let the speaker go on to long – brevity is a virtue!	*I hear what you are saying. Could you say it in just a sentence or two?*
Focus on the process: The point is to learn and practice skills – problems can be deferred to later sessions.	*That's a problem we can work on next week when we do problem solving. Right now, let's make sure we really understand each other.*

of the steps, it is often useful to have the child present/ready the handout and then go over it with the information included below. This allows more engagement of the family and child in the process. As noted, each step in the process has a rationale related to the overall concept:

Last week we talked about how the way we talk to each other can help to turn downward spirals into upward spirals. One of the important ways to start upward spirals is to tell other people in the family when we thought they did something well, were nice, or had a good idea. We call this "saying what you liked." When somebody tells us what they like about us, it feels good. Here's one way to say what you liked that really seems to work.

The first thing to do is to look at the person. This is important because then the person knows we're talking to them and that we mean what we say.

The next thing is to say exactly what they did that pleased you. When we do this, the person knows for sure what you liked and can do it again in the future.

The last thing is to tell them how it made you feel. When you tell them how it made you feel then they really know why you liked it.

Does this sound right?

> **Positive feedback practicing includes both silly and realistic role play examples**

Here we introduce role-playing, which can be challenging for some family members. By approaching the material slowly, starting with material that is less personal and moving toward more personal, relevant material, the therapist can build comfort in family members and increase the likelihood that the experience is more enjoyable for the child and parents/caregivers:

OK, now we'll do some practicing. One of the things we like to do in this treatment is to role-play. It's sort of like acting. Let's try it and see how it feels. In this box I have some pieces of paper and each one has written on it something someone could do or say or just something about them. Let's pretend it's about someone in the family who did each of these things and we'll practice telling each other that we liked it.

The giving positive feedback game (see Appendix 3) was designed with younger children in mind, and the items used in this game can be altered or updated in any way needed for older youth. We have found that if one does the silly items very tongue in cheek and with some eye-rolling, older youth enjoy it as well. The following is an example of a potential conversation:

We all need to watch carefully to make sure the person saying what they liked does everything on the sheet. We can give out tokens when someone does a good job and says what they liked in a good way. Remember to use the steps in the Saying What You Liked handout!

Give all family members about five tokens. The therapist should be the first to draw from the box and model the desired behavior. Play it out, and then get feedback on what was correct, frequently referring back to the handout. When family members give good feedback on the role-play, reward them with a token. Family members should then be encouraged to try the game. If family members seem enthusiastic, take a volunteer for the first role-play. If family members are hesitant, ask a parent to try out the role-play. Each therapist can construct their own box of items that can be changed to be developmentally appropriate for each child. Examples from our work include, "I liked it when you went bowling in your pajamas. It made me feel ____" and "I liked it when you helped me with my practice. It made me feel ____". This exercise should be lighthearted. By including both humorous and realistic examples in the box, family members may be more able to relax and engage in this game. The more practice in session, the better. The family can then be coached to use the items from their own list of upward spirals to give one another positive feedback about the real events of the week.

Starting with the parental dyad, or the therapist and parent, may put the child at ease and provide modeling: Ask the child to be a coach to make sure both do it right. Provide family members with lots of positive feedback on their skills, to provide both reinforcement and modeling of the desired behavior. When family members have difficulty, normalize the challenges of taking on a new behavior. Table 9 lists some challenges and suggestions for engaging in role-playing.

At the end of session give families additional tokens and assign the Keeping Upward Spirals Going (Handout 7) homework with praise for all their hard work.

Active Listening

Listening is framed as another important skill both for keeping upward spirals going and for stopping downward spirals. Family members are provided with Handout 8 describing the skill, and each step is carefully reviewed with the rationale for each clearly laid out:

The first thing to do is to look at the speaker: This way they know you are listening.

The second thing is to listen carefully: This way you can make sure you really hear what they say.

The third thing is to nod your head or say "uh-huh," then they know you're getting what they're saying.

The fourth thing is to ask questions if you are confused.

The last thing is to check out what you heard. When you do that, you can make sure you got it right.

During active listening, as in giving positive feedback, the therapist needs to take gradual steps, introducing the skill and then applying it to more personal and emotionally laden situations. First, practice with nonaffective content, emphasizing that in listening actively we must attend carefully to content. We have developed a game that uses made-up, often silly, examples for family members to use for active listening exercises (Appendix 3). For example, the speaker might be asked to briefly describe how to make a peanut butter and jelly sandwich. The listener can practice asking questions for clarification:

How about we play Let's Play It Out with this one? Ok, what I want you do is this. Let's have you [child] be the speaker and you [parent] be the active listener. Ok speaker, your job is to briefly tell your mom/dad exactly how you would make an ice cream sundae. [Parent], your job is to be a good active listener and do all the things on this Active Listening handout. You should be such a good listener that at the end you will know how to make a sundae just the way [child] told you to.

Second, practice with affective content, but use examples of others' feelings (role-play someone else). Here we emphasize that disclosures can sometimes involve important feelings that need to be acknowledged. For example, the speaker might be asked to describe how a child felt when they were benched during a game or when they won a prize on field day; the listener can practice reflecting the feelings:

Our job as a listener is even harder when the person talking is expressing their feelings. Sometimes by being a good listener we can help them with their feelings. We need to let them know we hear their feelings. So let's do it a little differently this time. This time [mom/dad] will be the speaker, and [child] will work on your active listening. So let's draw one of these cards and play it out. Oh, no, this person lost a $20 bill! Describe how it happened and how they felt about it.

It is often a good time for the therapist to take one of the roles and model the behavior first for the family, as reflecting affect can be a difficult skill for some participants. If the listener does not reflect back accurately, ask the speaker to verify that the reflection was accurate. If not, praise the effort, and try it again:

Did your [mom/dad] get it right? Is that really what you were trying to say?

Well, it sounds like you were really close, but it's important to be right on. So, let's try it again so we can make sure we got it right. After all, these skills take a lot of practice. It's not easy to be a good listener or to tell people just what we mean to say.

Third, and finally, we want to practice with real and personal examples to help family members to use the skill to actively attend to one another's feelings and to promote affective disclosure. Throughout, it is also important to let the speaker know that no one can listen and remember if we talk for too long (briefer exchanges are better). These exercises involving personal affective elements do not need to be heavy and painful – they can also involve situations of success and/or excitement. It's often good to start with rather innocuous examples like "describe a time you got a great birthday gift":

You're doing a great job on your listening skills and on telling each other about experience and giving each other information. Now let's practice telling one another about our real experiences and feelings and giving one another a chance to show good active listening. So I have these other cards, take one and let's practice. Maybe I'll do one to start and [mom/dad] you can be the listener. Sound good?

> **Families progressively practice listening skills, with non-emotional, emotional, and real family content**

Therapist would then choose an example from the envelope/bowl/hats and model a personal example and ask the parent to take the listener role, asking everyone else to coach using the Active Listening handout. For example, the item drawn might say "describe a time you felt scared and what it was like for you?" and a parent might be chosen to be the listener:

One time I was bike riding and I got on a hill that was too steep. I was really afraid I was going to get hurt going down that hill, but I couldn't turn around. I just had to go slowly but was scared all the way. My stomach was in quite a knot!

The parent can then go through each of the active listening steps on this simple example. The therapist then invites family members to take turns picking the items and doing the role-plays.

After families have enhanced their positive interactions and worked on their listening skills, the alliance between the therapist and the family, and particularly the child, is strengthened. At this point the focus can more easily shift to problems, as the family members have greater faith in the therapist's ability to help them and contain difficult emotions. Introducing the topic of giving negative feedback is a delicate one and should be clearly tied to the core treatment goal of decreasing downward spirals and increasing upward spirals. We often begin this briefly at the end of a positive communication session by asking families to come up with examples during the week:

One of the most important things with communication is to be able to identify problems early. Then we can use our active listening skills to help us talk with one another more helpfully so that we can stop downward spirals. So you know how we worked on catching upward spirals? Well, we want you to work on catching downward spirals this week. Next week, we'll use this to help us to stop those nasty spirals. So your home practice will be catching downwards spirals [Handout 9]. All families have downward spirals. Our job is to identify them and send them upward. We'll be working on this. Don't forget to give away all your tokens before next session! Good work today!

Introducing Giving Negative Feedback

Although the session on giving negative feedback is a full one, doing a few role-plays of positive feedback at the beginning of the session accomplishes two additional goals. First, it sets a positive tone at the outset: This is particularly important at this time as family members will now be working on giving some negative feedback. Second, it provides families with additional communication skills practice that they can then transfer to a new communication exercise – Saying What You Didn't Like (Handout 10). Crucially, the new skill needs to be tied to the core treatment goals and rationale:

> Even negative feedback sessions should start with positive feedback

We've been working on starting those upward spirals and keeping them going. By "saying what you liked" and using "active listening" you can help with those upward spirals. But sometimes you have a downward spiral starting, and it's important to stop it, for example, if someone is doing something not very nice. If you get mad and yell, it only makes the downward spiral keep going. So it's important to work on ways to help let other people know what they are doing that is upsetting you. Here's one way we do it. We call it "saying what you didn't like."

It is important to use reframing and normalizing here. For example, emphasizing that family members may do things to upset us or hurt our feelings without meaning to (reframing the intentions) and that in all relationships people do things that someone else sometimes does not like or wished they had done differently (normalizing). Treating this discussion with levity is important. The specific steps of the skill should then be reviewed:

> Therapists model and provide ongoing feedback on skill development

The first thing to do, just like with saying what you did *like, is to look at the person. You want them to know you are serious. The next thing is to say exactly what they did that you didn't like. Remember to keep looking at them. We need to be really clear about just what it was so they won't be confused: Be really specific! You then tell them how it made you feel. Then we give a suggestion for what they can do in the future. Does this make sense?*

Do a role-play, using a very innocuous example (i.e., forgetting to take out the trash or to put the cap back on the toothpaste). Make sure to point out the importance of being specific. For example, referring to the bedroom as a big mess is not as specific as noting the clothes on the floor, the apple cores on the shelf, and the unmade bed. Starting by drawing examples from the Let's Play It Out role-play game helps family members to practice the skill without jumping right into difficult personally relevant and potentially painful examples (see Appendix 3). Use tokens to reward a communication job well done and make family members monitor to make sure the speaker is doing all the items on the Saying What You Didn't Like handout.

As with other communication skills, the therapist should model first. Family members can then take turns trying. The items in the game are innocuous, sometimes even funny (in an eye-rolling way). Examples from our work include silly ones: "I don't like it when you put the dog in the dishwasher. It makes me feel ____. Next time wash him with a hose." And more serious ones: "I don't like it when you let others use my phone without my permission. It makes me feel ____. Next time, please ask my permission first." Making this lighthearted at first helps children to participate. Sometimes family members give commentary or moral lessons or accusations rather than saying how it makes them feel. Remind them to focus on feelings. It is important to remind family members that saying what you did not like may not solve the problem or guarantee others will not be angry/frustrated/disappointed: The goal is to improve communication around difficult issues so they may be more readily solved.

> Reframing angry exchanges and normalizing negative events in families is essential

Now try, delicately, to elicit family generated examples. This needs to be controlled carefully to not end up as an all-out gripe session or an attack on any one person. It is good for each family member to express a concern and each family member to be the object of an expressed concern. For example, you may ask the father what was one thing he wished his wife had done differently during the week, one thing the mother wishes the child had done differently, one thing the child wishes the father had done differently. If there is a dyad where considerable criticism from one member to the other is frequent (e.g., father to child), avoid using that dyad. The goal here is to practice the skill in a low-stress environment to the degree possible. Problems that arise in session can be dealt with using the very same problem-solving strategies.

Homework should encourage practice of this skill in a controlled way. Assign the Stopping Downward Spirals exercise (Handout 11) and emphasize the need to continue to notice and work on the upward spirals and to use the tokens.

Module 3: Things We Do Affect How We Feel

This module is one to two sessions.

> **CBT goal:** Increase reinforcers in the child's environment.
>
> **FT goal:** Increase positive family interactions.

Review of Homework

As usual, start with reviewing homework, praise, normalize, and practice. Make sure to do one round of positive feedback. As with all activities and skills in FFT-CD, you want to tie fun-activities planning (behavioral activation) to the treatment rationale – a way that we increase upward spirals and decrease downward spirals. Have family members write their ideas down on the Fun Activities handout (Handout 12), including the activity, who's included, how often they do it, and how much fun it is (Likert scale). Ask family members to share what is on their list with one another. Give tokens. The following is an example of a potential conversation:

Last week we talked about how the way we talk to each other can stop downward spirals by saying what you didn't like. We've also talked about saying what you liked to start upward spirals.

Doing fun things can also make a downward spiral turn upward. What are some fun things to do alone? Everybody probably has some different ideas. Let's all try to think of at least one thing that is fun to do by yourself and write it down.

There are fun things we can do by ourselves like the things you wrote down, and fun things we can do with friends, like going to a game or playing ball, and fun things we can do as a family, like going to the movies or playing a board game.

This brainstorming should be guided by several considerations. First, emphasize activities that are easily accessible with regard to cost, time, and distance. Children may put ideas for big ticket items – trips to theme parks – on this list: While these can certainly be included, developing a range of readily available activities is crucial. Playing a card game, throwing a ball, walking the dog, or spending time with a pet, spending 10 minutes drawing together – all are excellent options for many families. Second, use the list to enhance coping in a daily way. By including activities that the child can do when alone, with family, and friends, a wide range of coping options becomes available. Third, brainstorm fun activities that serve many functions. Activities can be enjoyable for different reasons – some allow us to enjoy time with others, some because they give us a feeling of mastery. All these are important:

> Families work together to list fun activities to do alone, with friends, and with family members

Some things are fun because they let us enjoy being with other people, and some are fun because they make us feel like we've done a good job – like drawing a really good picture or building something special. Let's all try to think of a few things that are fun to do as a family and write them down.

Although unusual, some families may have difficulties coming up with ideas for fun activities. In this case refer them to the Ideas for Fun Activities handout (Appendix 2).

Having produced a fun activities list, family members can then practice a new activity – Asking for What You Want (Handout 13). The goal here is to encourage family members to ask one another to engage in enjoyable activities. As with other activities, it should start by tying it to the core concept of interactional spirals:

Remember last week we talked about giving positive feedback and active listening? Yeah?

Well, another thing that can start a positive spiral is asking someone in the family for something in a nice way. We call this "asking for what you want."

The first thing to do is to look at the person, then they know they need to pay attention.

Second, it is important to say exactly what you want them to do. If you just say "be nice" or something like that, then they're not sure what to do.

Third, tell them how it would make you feel. When you tell them how it would make you feel, then they know why it is important.

Start by using the family games – pick an example out of the box/hat/ envelope and role-play it. Try to start the next exercise with a volunteer. If someone volunteers, give them a token and praise their willingness to try something new. After they pick the example from the box, ask to whom they

> Using tokens, families can be encouraged to try new activities together

would like to give the feedback. Have the other family members evaluate both what was good and what could be improved. Remind the family members to make sure the speaker covers all steps of the handout. After they have had a chance to practice using the game, move to the real family list and have them make requests to one another to engage in fun activities:

So it seems like we're getting pretty good at this. Let's try something a little different. You each have a list of fun things to do as a family. Let's practice making positive requests to do some fun things together. Remember the listener has to do active listening!

Start the practice with a different dyad than started the previous week. Have other family members act as coaches – making sure they start by noting the things about the communication exercise that went well. If they have difficulty, praise the aspects on which they did well, give a token for that, and have them try it again. At some point it is important to remind family members that using the communication training skills will not guarantee compliance:

One thing to remember about asking for what you want is that you won't always get it. You'll probably get it more often than if you ask in a way that isn't as nice, but not always. The important thing though is to talk to each other in a respectful way that makes everybody more comfortable at home.

For homework, decide on at least two fun things for the week (keep them small and make sure that each family member will likely enjoy the activity). Ask them to complete the Fun Things to Do sheet (Handout 14) prior to the next session.

Module 4: We Can Solve Problems Together

Families learn how solving problems can stop downward spirals

This module is three to four sessions and includes a number of pieces. It is often useful to divide the time as follows: one session for defining and specifying problems, one session for the emotional thermometer, one session for introducing problem solving, and one session for practicing problem solving. This division of time is flexible and should be tailored for each family's skill level and areas of need. For example, if a family is really able to understand the material quickly, problem definition and emotional thermometer can be done in one session: However, for a family with significant mood dysregulation, more than one session may need to be spent on the emotional thermometer and one problem-solving session may need to be focused on what to do when problems are too "hot" to handle.

Problem Identification

> **CBT goal:** Have each member of the family develop problem identification skills and practice self-monitoring of emotional states.
>
> **FT goal:** Reframe family problems as choices and opportunities to problem solve.

In our work with pre- and early adolescents a number of common problems emerge repeatedly, including setting limits for device use (internet access, smartphone use, social media), managing activities (crazy schedules, overwhelming demands), completing homework, sibling conflict, conflicts with extended family, peer conflicts, negotiating safety in the community, chores. The conflicts can appear to contribute to the core downward spirals that seem linked to the depression or to the overall stress environment: Either way, they provide opportunities to problem solve.

Problem Definition

This approach has been influenced by the work of Greene and Ablon on collaborative problem solving (Greene & Ablon, 2005). This model makes clear that problems can emerge as a function of competing needs. For example, the child wants to attend an event, but the parent's work schedule makes it impossible to take them. By framing this as a conflict in needs, the clinician can help open the door to a more collaborative approach with a number of potentially workable solutions, rather than as a parental yes/no decision. The goal is a win–win. The needs of both (or all) need to be attended for the problem to be solved adequately. In addition, problem solving can be done in a preventive way (optimal) or on an emergency basis (less optimal).

There are several goals in this section of problem solving. The first goal is to provide the link to the broader treatment rationale of reducing downward spirals:

We've been talking a lot about stopping downward spirals and turning them into upward spirals. We talked about giving each other positive feedback and doing fun things together. But what happens when you have a problem? Problems, when they don't get solved, can really lead to downward spirals. By knowing when you have a problem and working to find a good solution, you can stop those downward spirals.

The second goal is to get a sense of the range of problems. If parents/caregivers have completed the issues checklist (Robin & Weisz, 1980) at the outset of treatment, this can be revisited at this time. Given that children at this age are reluctant to acknowledge problems, it is useful at the outset to reframe a problem as a choice. Limited and innocuous self-disclosure can be useful here in normalizing problems:

Does your family have any problems? Of course! Everyone in every family has some problems or difficult situations each day. Mom has some of her own problems, Dad has some of his and [child] has some of theirs. And there can also be problems and situations at home that involve more than one person in the family. But the one thing all families have to do is to face their problems and cope with them, every day. With any problem you have choices. You have choices about how you are going to solve the problem. But first you have to know what the problem is. For example, I wanted to go to the movies last weekend, but I had to do the laundry. I had a problem.

To encourage the family to generate some examples of problems, the therapist can start in other settings, like work or school, and this may limit the initial stressfulness of this discussion. It is useful to write them on the board. Make sure each family member can give one or two examples, as it is important for children to see that parents/caregivers too have difficulties. There should be an attempt to be lighthearted here. Make observations (e.g., "it sounds like it can be really hard to keep things organized at work") and normalize (e.g., "with all the other expectations, it's not easy for kids these days to get all the practice done on time"). Problem examples should be specific, understandable to the child (at their level), and day to day. Complex parent problems (e.g., difficulties at work) may need to be translated into something the child can understand (e.g., "sometimes you have trouble getting your boss to listen to what you are saying"). The goal is to build skills in problem identification and problem solving. It is often necessary to help family members break problems down into manageable units (e.g., "sounds like there are several problems here").

The third goal is to practice using communication skills to define problems in solvable ways. We can ask each of the family members to use "saying what you didn't like" to communicate their point of view. One of the major stumbling blocks in problem solving is not agreeing on the nature of the problems. Defining Problems (Handout 15) gives instructions in problem definition and the What's the Problem? (Handout 16) can be completed to help families specify problems. Table 10 describes some of the potential problems,

Table 10
Rules for Problem Solving

Potential problems	Suggestions	Examples
Heated personal criticism/attacks.	Establish a "no blaming or name calling" rule.	*Although it may feel good in the moment to get angry and blame, this usually keeps the problem from getting solved. Sometimes we need to wait until the problem isn't so hot.*
Vague, unsolvable problems.	Be specific and behavioral: Break a complex problem down into manageable bits.	*Vague problems, like saying someone isn't nice, aren't easy to solve. We need to know exactly what the person is doing when they're not nice.*
Family members talk at length about history of the problem.	Keep it short and sweet.	*When people go on and on, other people tend to tune out or just think it's an impossible problem.*
An important player is missing (e.g., sibling, grandparent).	Ensure to know who's involved; invite for one or two problem-solving sessions.	*If a person who's really contributing to the problem isn't there, it's not likely you'll solve it without them.*
Family members are uncertain about their goal.	Hone in on what change is really needed and define "success" for this particular problem.	*It's also good to think about how things would be different if we get the problem solved. How would we know it was really solved?*

provides suggestions, and offers language for addressing them. Reviewing and normalizing these with the family prior to the move to addressing real family issues can ease that process:

When the problem includes more than one person in the family, it's important to solve the problem together. We talked about some problems you all have in your lives: How about in the family? What are some problems in your family? In some families doing practice can be a problem, or bedtimes can be a problem, or feeding the pets. Everyone write down three things that can sometimes be a problem at your house. In all families there are some big problems and some smaller ones. Let's think of some of each.

The fourth goal is to help family members determine who should be involved in solving the problems. Many problems do not get solved because a crucial participant is missing. We frequently include family members in some sessions to address particular problems. For example, our experience suggests, unsurprisingly, that sibling conflict can be a frequent source of downward spirals. Inviting siblings to attend one or two sessions to work on solving problems can be very instructive. In addition, differentiate problems that are *family* problems and those that are not and ask them to give examples:

> Some problems are best solved by the child alone, others with family involvement

When you have a problem, sometimes you want to solve it on your own and sometimes you need some help. Can you think of some problem you'd rather solve on your own? Sometimes it's important to let our family know when we have a problem we want to solve on our own and that they need to give us some time by ourselves to do it. One way to let them know is to make a positive request. Let's try it.

Practice using a positive request. Have the child practice asking to handle a problem on their own. It is especially important to have the child practice this skill, as appropriate assertiveness may be deficient in depressed children.

Taking Emotional Temperature

Using an emotional thermometer is a regular procedure in many evidence-based interventions, particularly when addressing anxiety concerns. In this context it is focused on helping families regulate the conflict by recognizing feelings and reactions to problems. In considering the family context several steps are important. First, families need to recognize how strong emotions can get in the way of problem solving:

> An emotional thermometer worksheet can be used to identify "cooler" problems for initial practice

When there's a problem sometimes people in the family get upset, but it's not too good to try solving problems when you are too upset, because this can lead to downward spirals.

Second, the Emotional Thermometer handout (Handout 17) can be used to introduce this idea. The more examples the better. We include one such example in Figure 5. Have each family member rate a few problems on their list to get the hang of it. Third, relate emotional temperature to the problem of selecting problems for problem solving and consider how family members help themselves to cool off and be ready to solve a problem:

When we first start working on problem solving, it is good to try to solve some easier ones, the ones that don't get your emotional temperature too high. That way we can get some good practice in and be ready for the bigger problems. Everybody

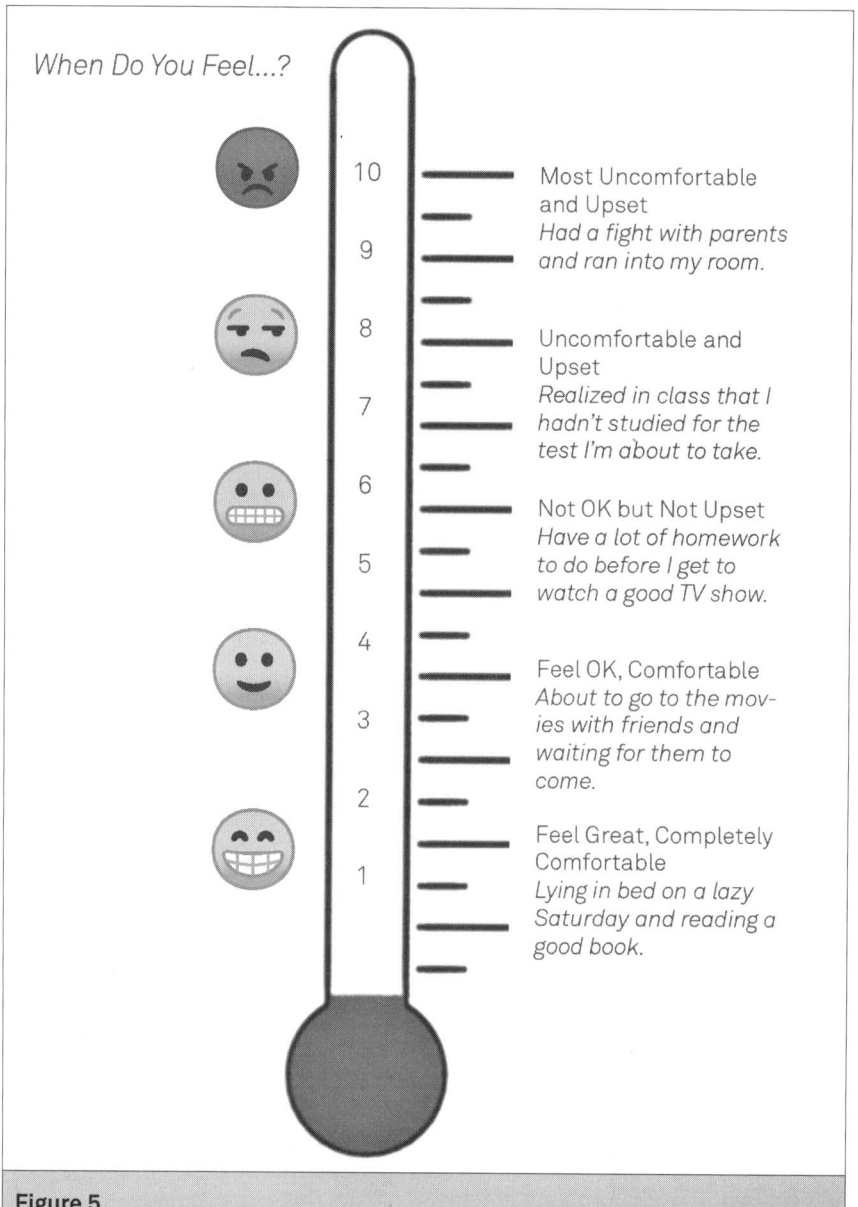

Figure 5
Sample emotional thermometer. A blank version is available in Handout 17.

does different things to try to feel better when they get upset about a problem. How about you?

One caution is that it is easy for the child to become the target during these sessions. A couple of strategies can be used to reduce this risk: Choose problems that do not focus on the child for some of the problem-solving exercises (especially at the beginning), including nonfamily problems, and choose an imminently solvable problem at the outset to help families work on skills. Families may get frustrated if the problems they view as most vexing are not addressed. It is often helpful to acknowledge these difficult problems and note that you will work on them during therapy (e.g., "it sounds like the issue of people not working together at home is a tough one, and we are going to get to that one").

Homework/Practice

Assign the task of each family member recording a few problems daily this week and specifying which are individual and which are family problems. Have them take their emotional temperature for each problem and determine whether it is an individual or family problem using Handout 16. Also, make sure that they continue to use their tokens throughout the week to maintain a positive focus while also addressing difficult issues.

Problem-Solving Model

> **CBT goal:** Skills training and practice in conflict resolution skills.
> **FT goal:** Empower family to solve and become more flexible in approaching problems.

Strategies in the session include picking a problem to solve, taking the temperature for this problem, presenting the problem-solving model, and implementing the problem-solving model. The first two steps were discussed in the previous session and can be practiced here. If the temperature on particular problems is too high, select one that is a little cooler so that problem-solving skills can be more readily practiced. Pick one that is mentioned by more than one person and is not too difficult. Pick one that is likely to involve a more peripherally involved member to engage them in the process. The goal is to practice problem-solving skills as a family. At this point it is important that, to the degree possible, those who are involved in the problem be included in the problem-solving process.

In some families, mood regulation is a central problem. This quickly becomes apparent during the description of the downward spirals and may make introduction of the emotional thermometer tricky. Sometimes these families will report that all of their problems have an emotional temperature of 100 plus. In these families, the therapist needs to make a judgment about whether to move to particular problems or to initially focus problem solving on mood regulation in general:

In more volatile families, therapists can focus on problem solving about mood regulation

It sounds like in your family sometimes it's hard to cool down enough to solve the problems. Maybe one problem we need to work on is helping the family find ways to cool off a bit before talking about the problem itself.

The problem-solving model is then introduced using Solving Problems (Handout 18) with careful review of each step:

First you have to agree on the problem, because if you don't agree on what the problem is then you can't work to solve it.

Second, everyone suggests some possible solutions. Everybody needs to give their ideas here. It's like brainstorming. Don't throw ideas away yet: After all, what seems like a dumb idea at first might turn out to be the best idea of all!

Third, the family has to discuss the good parts and bad parts of each idea and then pick the one that seems like the best. Sometimes it's a couple of solutions put together.

Fourth, everybody needs to agree on a plan to carry out the solution.

Finally, when you've tried it, you have to go over it again to see whether it worked and decide to change it if needed.

At this point, have the family work on the problem-solving issue that they have chosen. Use the longer Problem Solving Worksheet (Handout 19) to give families more room to write ideas down. There are some cautions to keep in mind with families at each step of the problem-solving model. In defining the problem, use the previous sessions' lessons. In suggesting possible solutions, the therapist should emphasize the brainstorming nature of the task and stop family members from prematurely discarding potential solutions. The family should be reminded that they will have an opportunity to evaluate all solutions during the next phase and that sometimes a silly solution turns out to be the best one in the end. At times to emphasize this point, and to add humor to the interaction, the therapist may try to suggest one outlandish solution and emphasize the importance of not dismissing it – all potential solutions should be evaluated! It is important that each family member contribute to this process, as everyone needs to be invested in finding a solution. However, limiting the total number of solutions (no more than five per problem) will be necessary to allow time for evaluation of them all.

> **Problem solutions often don't work the first time and must be honed over time**

In discussing pros and cons (for youth we use "pluses" and "minuses") of each potential solution, all solutions should be evaluated as the best solution may often be a combination of the suggestions. Contingency contracting (in which one family member agrees to change their behavior in exchange for change in another family member) may be particularly useful in demonstrating the necessity of compromise. In planning and carrying out the chosen solution, make sure to include the date and time of implementation, the responsibilities of each party, any needed resources and who will obtain them, and anticipate what might go wrong. The therapist will need to make certain each family member understands the solution and their role in it. After completion, praise efforts and review how it worked. It is useful to predict that the problem solution will not work perfectly. (If problems are too easy to solve they are not really problems!) Many problems will not be solved fully and satisfactorily on the first attempt (and this should be emphasized for family members). Given that family problems may be long-standing, it is important to lower expectations and recognize that they will take time to figure out, and the first solution may not be the final one.

After implementation of the solution, it is essential to review its effectiveness and to renegotiate where necessary. However, family members should be praised and learn to praise one another for their attempts to make a change. During this process core downward spirals can be identified. What are the conflicts that keep coming up? These are often the heart of the treatment. Spelling out how these repeatedly negatively impact the child and family can lead to greater communication and allow for a problem solution that will impact numerous situations. For example, in one case the child would push the mother away when she was emotionally dysregulated and then feel lonely and abandoned while her mother would leave the situation and feel helpless and ineffectual. After identifying this spiral and the sad feelings it evoked in both family members, we were able to engage in communication exercises to enhance understanding of its precipitants, process, and outcome and then use the problem-solving exercise to come up with a mutually agreed-upon strategy to help them address the child's emotional dysregulation more effectively. These interventions achieved the goal of increasing the child's coping skills (e.g., enhanced assertiveness, self-reflection) and improved the parent–child relationship (e.g., enhanced communication and understanding of how to help one another navigate difficult interactions).

There are a number of cautions to consider in family-based problem solving. First, solutions that involve more than one family member to change are likely to be more effective. One-person solutions reinforce the identified patient concept, tending to blame that individual for ongoing difficulties. If you have difficulty getting away from problems that require change from only one person, then find other problems to work on that will require change from other family members. Second, stay focused on the present situation and stop any attempts to dredge up old examples of similar problems. The focus should be on what is to be done in the here and now. Avoid getting sidetracked. Third, work on one problem at a time. One specific problem is more likely to be solved and less likely to go off track. Using the communication skills may help focus and define the problem in a more behavioral way.

Applying solutions to specific problems can allow families to identify core conflicts

Homework

Implement the problem solution. As always make sure the positives keep going with tokens to and from each family member. Family members report back at the next session and evaluate success.

Module 5: Saying Goodbye

This module focuses on therapy termination and relapse prevention and includes one to two sessions.

> **CBT goal:** Additional practice in problem solving and encouraging generalization of skills.
> **FT goal:** Establish a family meeting time and commitment to increase positive interactions and establish better family problem resolution.

Problem-Solving Ongoing Change

At this point families should be fairly adept at implementing the problem-solving approach. Present the problem that the family will no longer be in therapy:

These sessions are a place where your family can talk together, schedule fun things to do, give each other positive feedback, and solve problems. Even though you won't be coming here anymore, you still need to do all these things. Let's solve this problem together. How can you keep up our new skills without coming in for these sessions any longer?

This process should be lighthearted. As one problem solution the therapist should suggest a weekly meeting with specified goals of practicing communication, solving problems, and planning fun family and individual activities. Despite the end of therapy, booster sessions are available and the therapist can continue to be a resource for the family. Make referral for ongoing treatment as necessary.

Review Therapy

The child is presented with a booklet, which includes all the handouts that have been used over the course of treatment. This brightly colored booklet, typically bookended with construction paper, should include space on the cover for the child to print their name and add drawings should they choose. The rationale presented to the child is that the book is a resource (like the skills themselves) that can be used in the future when difficulties with mood arise. After giving the book to the child, open it up, go through each of the pages, remind the child and other family members of each skill you have worked on and how it relates back to the model.

Anticipate and Problem Solve Stressors

Acknowledge that there is always work to be done and that the family can use the skills they have been working on to keep progress going. Ask the family about stressors they anticipate facing in the next few months and do some anticipatory problem solving. Normative transitions are a frequent focus – starting middle school, going to a new summer camp, etc. Here is another place where normalizing is important – stress is a regular part of life and can be present even for positive, exciting events, and the family and child have developed skills to better manage it.

> **Final sessions include anticipating stressors and developing potential strategies to manage them**

4.3   Challenges in Implementing FFT-CD

Depression in youth is complicated to treat with its high comorbidity and frequent parental mental health challenges. To prominently address concerns the therapist may alter the order of the intervention models, as summarized in Table 11. Four particular challenges bear mentioning. First, in some cases of more severe depressive disorders, children may display serious anhedonia and low activity level. Here we start the treatment with a focus on behavioral activation. It is not always easy to identify pleasurable activities: Those activities that were once sources of pleasure provide a starting off point for these discussions. Second, children who have significant comorbidities may need additional intervention components. Problem solving may help to identify these concerns and strategize for additional resources (e.g., testing/evaluation, medication consultation, focused sessions on parent management). We have found that often times challenges associated with comorbidities can

Table 11
Special Challenges That May Influence the Order of Treatment Modules

Child/family characteristics	Change in module order	Goal
Anhedonia/ low activity	Start with behavioral activation/planning fun activities.	Increasing children's motivation to engage in treatment and work outside of session.
Externalizing comorbidity	Problem solving (a small, solvable problem); shift quickly to promoting positive interactions.	Increasing parent and child optimism about treatment.
High family conflict	Communication training or additional psychoeducation, sometimes including/ focusing on subsystem sessions.	Increasing awareness of the impact of conflict and enhancing skills to reduce it in the short term.
Family crisis/ child suicidality	Problem solving focused on the crisis situation or safety planning.	Stabilizing/resolving crisis, decreasing suicide risk.

fuel downward spirals and can become a central focus of communication and problem-solving work. The broad framing of FFT-CD makes it a useful strategy for addressing depression in the context of comorbidity. Third, severe family conflict can challenge implementation of any family-based treatment. Where interparental conflict is severe or parents/caregivers have a nonamicable relationship rupture (e.g., separation, divorce), additional sessions with parents/caregivers to focus on joint goals and communication can be useful: At times we have focused on conjoint sessions with each parent and child dyad and not attempted to have both parents/caregivers in one session. Parents/ caregivers can then be coached on out-of-session communication with one another to reduce stress on the child. Fourth, during a family crisis we may move directly into a problem-solving mode to address this situation at hand. Child suicidality can be one such crisis and is addressed in more detail next.

Although children with depression are at lower risk for suicide attempts and completed suicide than are adolescents with depression, evaluating and managing suicidal thoughts and behaviors is critical in implementing any treatment for depressive disorders (Pettit, Buitron, & Green, 2018). Our procedures for evaluating risk begin with our individual meeting with the child at the outset of each family session to assess symptoms, as this provides an opportunity to query about ideation and behavior on a weekly basis. The slightly expanded version of the Depression Self-Rating Scale (Asarnow & Carlson, 1985) includes items on thoughts of death and suicide to allow for regular screening. If a child endorses any of these items, we then follow up with additional evaluations to assess risk, including the Columbia Suicide

Severity Rating Scale (Posner et al., 2011) with information from both the child and parent. As in all risk management, the level of intervention is commensurate with the degree of risk. In our large randomized controlled trial, we had few incidents where suicidal ideation/plan necessitated evaluation in the Emergency Department.

In many ways, a family-based approach provides an ideal context for addressing risk concerns, as parents/caregivers are already engaged, and the model focuses on enhancing family support. In cases of new or increased suicidal risk, we usually move quickly to problem solving with a focus on safety planning. Family members can brainstorm and decide on plans to communicate risk level on a daily basis and to provide brief distracting activities to engage in when suicidal thoughts emerge. Individual time with parents/caregivers can focus on psychoeducation about suicide in youth, specific instructions for improving the safety of the home (e.g., securing firearms and other potentially dangerous items), and emergency plans. The foci of treatment, including building family communication and enhancing pleasurable activities, are in line with longer-term interventions focused on reducing suicide risk (Tompson et al., 2012).

4.4   Efficacy of FFT-CD

> Initial pilot work on FFT-CD underscored the need for flexibility

FFT-CD was developed in three stages – open trial pilot testing and treatment development, a small, randomized trial comparing it to a wait-list control, and a large trial comparing it to another active depression-focused intervention. In the open trial we collected feedback from families to develop our handouts and to design/test our strategies (Tompson et al., 2007). Through this early work, we learned lessons. First, given youth and parents/caregivers have busy lives, both parents/caregivers cannot always attend, and we had to be flexible and include sessions with parents/caregivers separately, together, and in other groupings. Second, we frequently had to include siblings. When families had very young siblings, including them in sessions was often necessary for both parents/caregivers to attend. By providing age-appropriate activities we found they could often be in the room during much of the session time. For families with other school-aged children, we found that sibling conflict could often precipitate downward spirals. By including siblings in at least some sessions we could enhance problem solving for the family more broadly. Third, although medication is considered one essential piece in many family-based interventions (e.g., FFT for bipolar disorders in youth), many parents/caregivers of depressed children preferred to focus on a psychosocial approach. For this reason, FFT-CD does not assume medication is a regular part of treatment for all youth. Where medications are used for either the depression or other associated problems (e.g., ADHD) problems with adherence can be a focus of problem solving.

The randomized clinical trial was completed at two sites – Boston University and University of California, Los Angeles – and compared

FFT-CD to individual psychotherapy (IP). IP was a manualized supportive, client-centered approach (based on Cohen and Mannarino, 1996) that stressed empathic listening, support, encouragement, and nondirective problem solving. Youth ages 7–14 years ($n = 134$) with diagnoses of MDD, dysthymic disorder (DD), or depression NOS participated in the trial. We included youth with comorbid anxiety and behavioral disorders but excluded youth with mental health and developmental disorders that might interfere with treatment or assessment (e.g., psychotic disorder, autism spectrum disorder, severe obsessive-compulsive disorder, active substance abuse/dependence, mental retardation, serious conduct disorder). At the baseline evaluation there was no differences between the groups on demographic variables (age, gender, race/ethnicity) or clinical characteristics (severity, chronicity, depression diagnosis, comorbid diagnoses, medication status, or history of treatment utilization).

Participants were randomly assigned to FFT-CD or IP on a 1:1 ratio and groups were balanced on site, gender, baseline depression diagnosis (MDD or DD versus depressive disorder NOS), and the presence versus absence of antidepressant medication treatment (only about 10% of the sample were taking these medications). The same therapists conducted both the FFT-CD and the IP interventions at each site. We implemented rigorous training and quality assurance procedures to ensure both interventions were delivered as specified in our treatment manuals (Tompson, Sugar et al., 2017; Asarnow et al., 2020). Participants were evaluated immediately posttreatment and at 4-month and 9-month follow-up points by raters who were blind to the treatment assignment. Children and their parents also completed the CDI at each of these assessment points and at the 5th and 10th treatment sessions: Additional information on study design and implementation can be found in our previous publications (Tompson, Sugar et al., 2017; Asarnow et al., 2020).

The primary outcome examined was adequate clinical depression response, defined as a decrease in the Children's Depression Rating Scale–Revised (CDRS-R) of ≥50%. Given the sparse literature on child depression treatment, we chose this outcome to be consistent with adolescent depression treatment trials (Tompson et al., 2012). In addition, we examined clinical depression remission, defined as a posttreatment CDRS-R score ≤28. We chose this outcome to be consistent with youth antidepressant treatment trials (Cipriani et al., 2016). We examined both immediate posttreatment outcomes as well as longer-term outcomes and response trajectories and used an intent-to-treat approach (including those who dropped out of treatment early and did not complete assessment). As illustrated in Figure 6, FFT-CD children showed higher rates of adequate clinical depression response immediately following treatment than did IP children, and this was true when we included dropouts in our analyses or focused only on those who completed treatment. Almost 80% of those in FFT-CD responded, compared to 60% in IP. We saw a similar picture for depression remission. However, the degree of change on the overall CDRS-R score did not differ between groups, as there was significant variability within both groups. Consistent with our expectations, the advantages of FFT-CD were most evident for younger youth: Those

> Children assigned to FFT-CD showed greater treatment response than children assigned to individual psychotherapy

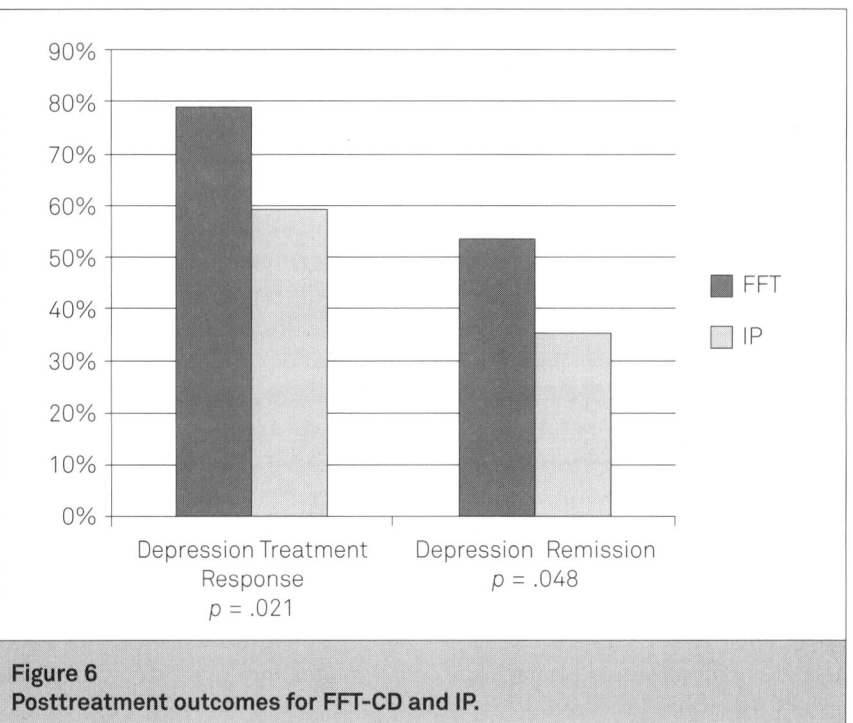

Figure 6
Posttreatment outcomes for FFT-CD and IP.

aged 7–11 years had an odds ratio for adequate depression clinical response of almost 3:1 favoring FFT-CD while those aged 12–14 years had an odds ratio of roughly to 1:1 across the two treatment conditions. It appears that FFT-CD may be most beneficial during the childhood years but comparable to IP as youth enter adolescence. This supports our contention that FFT-CD is a developmentally appropriate and targeted intervention.

Examining longer-term effects and trajectories, we followed children for 52 weeks, roughly 9 months after treatment completion (Asarnow et al., 2020). We were able to use data collected at each of our follow-ups, as well as data collected during the treatment (Weeks 5 and 10) using the child- and parent-reported depressive symptoms on the CDI (CDI-C and CDI-P). With this longitudinal model with six time points, FFT-CD showed a significant advantage over IP on the CDI-C during the acute treatment period and an overall trend for differential trajectories across groups. In both groups there was significant initial improvement in symptoms, followed by a leveling off over the follow-up. For the CDI-P, both treatment groups showed significant initial gains, followed by leveling off over the follow-up.

Across diverse depression measures (CDRS response, total score, remission), we observed a consistent pattern of greater improvement in depression levels among youth receiving FFT-CD at the posttreatment point. However, over the follow-up period (posttreatment assessment through Week 52), children assigned to IP continued to gradually improve and those assigned to FFT-CD leveled out. Indeed, most children recovered from their depressive episodes by Week 52 (roughly 12 months): 77% in FFT-CD, 78% IP. Despite the relatively short follow-up period, some youth had recurrent episodes that also emerged including one in FFT-CD and six in IP; survival analyses revealed a trend toward an FFT-CD advantage in preventing recurrence.

We also evaluated suicidal behavior, self-harm, mental-health-related Emergency Department visits, and psychiatric hospitalizations (Asarnow et al., 2020) over the course of this clinical trial. In terms of suicidal behavior, four children made five suicide attempts (one hanging, two overdoses, one cutting, one method unknown) and all were assigned to IP (one during treatment and four during Weeks 16–52). In terms of nonsuicidal self-injury, this was reported for 15 children, with seven in FFT-CD (six children for 15 episodes during treatment, one child for one episode during Weeks 16–52) and eight in IP (six children for 12 episodes during treatment, five children for nine episodes during Weeks 16–52). Emergency Department visits for mental-health-related concerns were similar across treatment groups with four FFT-CD children (two children with three total visits during treatment, two children with four total visits Weeks 16–52) and four IP children (two children with two total visits during treatment, two children with three total visits Weeks 16–52). There were few mental-health-related hospitalizations across the study with three FFT-CD children (two children with two total hospitalizations during treatment, one child with three total hospitalizations during Weeks 16–52) and two IP children (one during treatment, one during Weeks 16–52).

> **FFT-CD may reduce risk of suicidal behavior and depression relapse compared to IP**

These data are consistent with the few studies that have examined family-based treatments for mood disorders in youth. Dietz and colleagues (2015) compared a family-based interpersonal psychotherapy to client-centered therapy for 8–12-year-old children and found higher rates of remission, reduced anxiety, and improved interpersonal functioning in the family versus individual condition. Although similar in its interpersonal focus, the family-based therapy differed from FFT-CD in integrating more individual child sessions. Miklowitz and colleagues (2006) developed FFT for adolescents with bipolar disorder based on models that demonstrated efficacy among adults with bipolar disorder (Miklowitz et al., 2003; Rea et al., 2003): This intervention combined family psychoeducation and skills training to better manage bipolar disorder. In a series of studies, they compared this FFT to enhanced care (three sessions of family psychoeducation) as an adjunct to mood-stabilizing medications for bipolar disorders in youth (ages 12–18 years) and found mixed support. In the first study (Miklowitz et al., 2008), those in FFT showed more rapid recovery from the initial mood episode, lower risk of recurrence, and fewer mood symptoms in the two years following treatment. However, these results were not replicated in a larger trial (Miklowitz et al., 2014).

FFT-CD is a developmentally tailored and targeted intervention and, not surprisingly, appears to be particularly useful for children rather than adolescents. At the same time, in our clinical trial, young adolescents (up to age 14 years) responded positively to the intervention model with the vast majority demonstrating recovery during treatment. Much remains to be done to understand the mechanism by which family treatments exert their impact, and to identify predictors of who might benefit most from a family approach versus an individual approach.

5

Case Vignettes

This chapter describes the implementation of FFT-CD with three youth. In order to respect privacy and confidentiality, the cases described here are disguised and/or composites of actual cases. They illustrate the many challenges of treatment with a family-focused approach. First, each case has a different family situation, history, and functioning. Second, they come from different racial/ethnic and economic backgrounds. Third, they include a boy and two girls, across the ages of 7 to 12 years, both pre- and postpubertal. For each family the challenge is to use the framework and strategies of the FFT-CD approach while carefully tailoring to address each child and family's background, current situation, and interpersonal processes.

Case Vignette 1: Rebuilding the Mother–Child Relationship

The case of Leah is from "A Family-Based Approach to the Treatment of Youth Depression," by M. C. Tompson, C. Swetlitz, & J. R. Asarnow, in J. L. Allen, D. J. Hawes, & C. A. Essau (Eds.), *Family-Based Intervention for Child and Adolescent Mental Health* (pp. 87–99), 2021, Cambridge University Press. © 2021. Reprinted with permission of the licensor through PLSclear.

Initial Presentation

Leah was a 12-year-old Latina seventh-grade girl who presented with depressed mood, low self-esteem, suicidal ideation, and sleep disturbances. She lived with her mother and three younger siblings. Leah's mother and grandmother had a history of depression. However, Leah's mother was remarkably resilient. Although born into poverty and giving birth to Leah in high school, she was fully employed, maintained strong relationships with family and friends, and was effectively raising her three children alone. Although Leah's mother worked hard to provide for Leah and her siblings, finances remained a major source of familial stress. Although loving, Leah's father was inconsistently involved in her life. Leah, a bright girl and exceptional student, found refuge from these difficult circumstances in school. While Leah and her mother had once been very close, their relationship had eroded in the wake of these environmental stressors. Leah's mother expressed a longing to become close with her daughter again.

Early Phase of Treatment

Although Leah was open to participating in treatment, she doubted that her relationship with her mother would improve. She felt constantly criticized by her mother and tended to withdraw as a result. When Leah isolated herself, her mother would attempt to engage Leah by becoming harsh or intrusive with her, causing Leah to pull away even more. For example, Leah's mother would initiate discussion about sexuality. This was a principal concern of Leah's mother given her own unplanned pregnancy as a teenager. Leah was not comfortable discussing this topic with her mother and would withdraw when it was brought up. While this downward spiral (Figure 7) was readily identified by Leah and her mother during the One Way to Understand

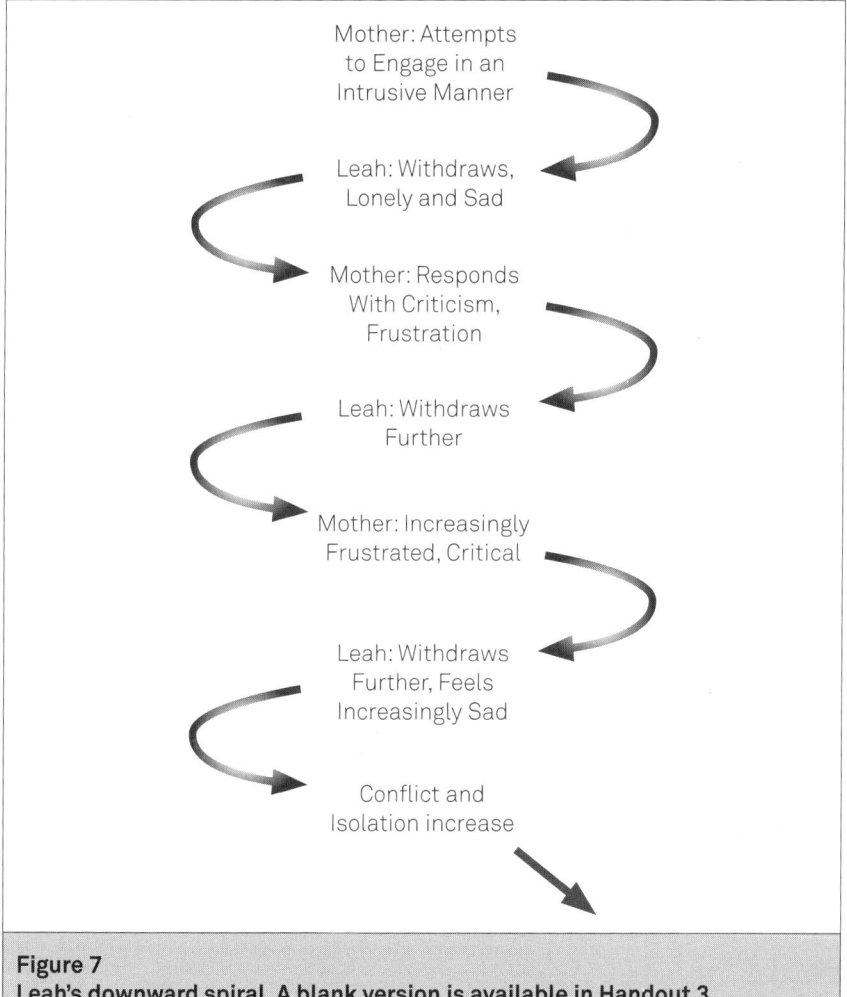

Figure 7
Leah's downward spiral. A blank version is available in Handout 3.

Depression module neither Leah nor her mother were able to offer examples of upward spirals.

Leah's initial resistance to treatment and tendency to withdraw continued into the beginning stages of the Families Talking Together module. When asked to give her mother some positive feedback, Leah withdrew and refused to role-play. The clinician responded to this by demonstrating ways that Leah could reinforce others' positive behavior and tried role-playing with Leah's mother. Similarly, Leah's mother became upset and used harsh language upon hearing negative feedback from Leah, prompting Leah to withdraw. The clinician helped Leah and her mother to identify this as the beginning of a downward spiral, and Leah's mother said that she would try to be mindful about her tone and levels of irritability when stressed.

Nonetheless, it was during this phase of treatment that treatment gains were first observed. Leah and her mother seemed to bond over the use of thanks notes and used humor to playfully ease tension around communication exercises at home. As Leah and her mother began to notice and acknowledge the small positives in their relationship, Leah's depressive symptoms began to subside. Leah began to spend more time outside her room and was finally able to acknowledge positive interactions with her mother.

Middle Phase of Treatment

The clinician decided to spend less time on the Things We Do Affect How We Feel module due to the emergence of a significant environmental stressor. Leah's family had to move out of their apartment, and Leah would have to switch schools as a result. This was devastating to Leah as school was a source of comfort and solace for her. Instead, the clinician introduced the We Can Solve Problems Together module and employed problem-solving strategies around finding an affordable apartment within the same school district. While there were obvious benefits to this solution, there were also downsides – in order to stay in the district, Leah's mother would need to work more hours and would have less time to spend with Leah. The clinician emphasized this as well. Interestingly, even with this stressor, Leah's depression symptoms continued to decrease. The clinician returned to the Things We Do Affect How We Feel module to continue stopping downward spirals and starting upward spirals.

Final Phase of Treatment

By the end of treatment, both Leah and her mother reported feeling more supported by the other, and Leah's depressive symptoms showed significant reductions. In one of their final sessions, Leah revealed to her mother that she was struggling with her sexual orientation. To this, Leah's mother expressed her unconditional and loving support. Given that conversations concerning sexuality were once a major source of tension between Leah and her mother, this interaction was an important milestone, both in their relationship and in

Leah's course of treatment. While Leah's depression emerged in the absence of preexisting psychopathology, it manifested during a period of elevated strain in a family struggling to break out of poverty. This stressful environment contributed to the erosion of a once supportive mother–daughter relationship – one that eventually became a stressor in itself. In this case, it was evident that enhancing communication between Leah and her mother was core to her symptom improvements. At discharge, Leah presented as a confident and capable early adolescent.

Case Vignette 2: Working With Depression in the Context of Anxiety

The case of Adele is from "Family-Focused Treatment of Childhood Depression: Model and Case Illustrations" by M. C. Tompson, D. A. Langer, J. L. Hughes, & J. R. Asarnow, 2017, *Cognitive and Behavioral Practice*, 24(3), pp. 269–287. © 2017 by Elsevier. Reprinted with permission from Elsevier.

Initial Presentation

Adele, a 9-year-old Italian-American girl, was in the third grade and lived with her parents and 4-year-old brother. She was diagnosed with double depression. According to Adele's parents, she had been "sensitive" and difficult to soothe as an infant, had experienced clinically impairing separation anxiety as young child, and, upon starting elementary school, demonstrated great anxiety about what to wear to school, resulting in frequent refusal to dress in the morning. Adele's parents recalled some symptoms starting during Kindergarten: low mood and irritability, difficulty sleeping (long latency to sleep and frequent nighttime waking), low self-esteem, and difficulty concentrating. They reported that during the last month, these symptoms worsened and new ones emerged, including lack of enjoyment of once fun activities, increased fatigue, decreased appetite, excessive guilt, and saying she wished she was "dead." Similarly, Adele reported feeling sad more days than not, especially at school, and thinking about things she would like to change about herself. She reported feeling guilty when another child was reprimanded, even though she had done nothing wrong. Though she thought things might get better, she was not able to articulate anything she was looking forward to. Mother's target problems included: concerns about Adele's safety, low self-esteem particularly during homework time, her unhappiness, and difficulties getting ready for school and the associated anxiety. Although anxiety is not necessarily a focus of FFT-CD, it often contributes to downward spirals and integration of anxiety-focused interventions may become a part of problem solving associated with reducing these downward spirals.

Early Phase of Treatment

Adele and her parents were highly motivated. Initial sessions focused on engaging the family and explaining the treatment rationale and plan. Although, typically, sessions focus on the depressed youth and her parents, due to a lack of child care the family was faced with the choice of having one of the parents stay home (or in the waiting room) with the brother or have him in the treatment room. In discussion with the therapist, the family decided to have him in the room, playing independently for some sessions and joining in when possible (e.g., handing out and receiving tokens). This allowed Adele to see how even with him present, her parents were able to focus primarily on her and work as a subsystem. Adele and her parents easily provided examples of downward and upward spirals during the psychoeducation module. Typically, a downward spiral would occur when getting ready in the morning (Figure 8) or doing homework in the afternoon. The therapist highlighted how, not by the fault

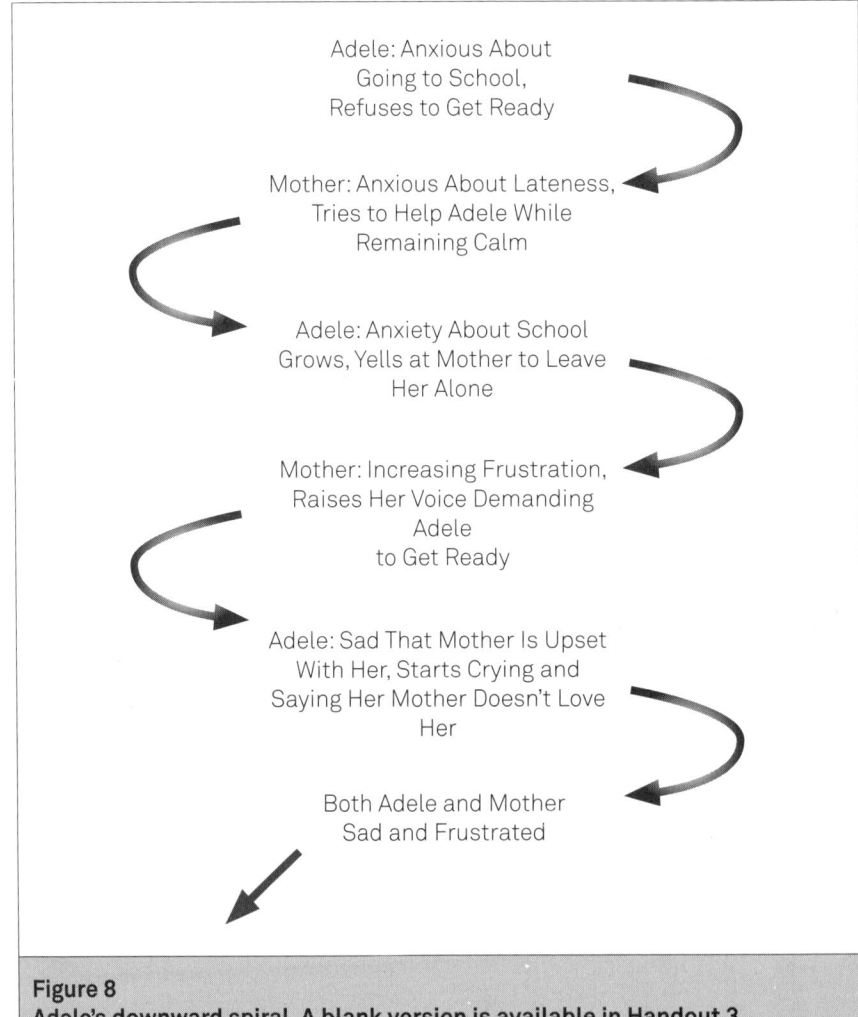

Figure 8
Adele's downward spiral. A blank version is available in Handout 3.

of anyone, each would respond to the other's stress by getting more stressed. Adele's parents noted that when they tried to support Adele, for example, with her difficulty putting on clothes in the morning, she would often become angrier with them. The therapist used this opportunity to normalize both downward and upward spirals, and note that the goal of treatment was to learn more effective ways to decrease (and stop) downward spirals and start (and maintain) upward spirals. In the session with Adele's parents alone, Adele's mother reported understanding Adele's symptoms because she had also suffered from depression. Although this increased her empathy, she also felt guilt, worrying that her own struggles with depression may have set up Adele for similar struggles.

Middle Phase of Treatment

This phase focused on communication and problem-solving skills, starting with increasing positivity by "saying what you liked." Adele's family picked up this skill easily and enjoyed giving tokens to one another for both real and made-up silly reasons. By the fourth session the family began working on active listening. As is common for many children and parents, giving cues that indicate active listening (e.g., nodding, saying "uh-huh") came more easily to Adele and her parents, though it took more practice for them to check out what they heard by repeating it back. Their default response was either to respond to the statement by providing their own opinions (instead of checking out what they heard first) or repeating back one aspect of what they heard while missing key points. Normalizing this challenge, the therapist used it as an example for the family of the importance of checking out what is heard, as, even when people think they have listened carefully, it is easy to miss things (and, for parents, it is best to keep statements short if they want their child's full attention). After covering the "saying what you didn't like" skill, the family used their communication skills to discuss the downward spiral that occurred around getting dressed for school. For the bulk of the session, Adele and her parents alternated speaking and listening roles. A parent would say what was disliked in the morning and what was preferred, and Adele would actively listen and check out what she heard. Upon confirmation that she heard the parent's statement accurately (sometimes with a few attempts), she would share her opinion and parents would actively listen. Through this iterative process, each expressed their needs and preferences, and they agreed on a plan to attempt, which, with only minor tweaking in following weeks, was successful.

Building off the success of communication skills for solving a problem, the therapist and family moved on to the problem-solving modules to learn how to solve problems collaboratively when good communication alone was not sufficient. After practicing with made-up and less emotionally heated problems, the family tackled the problem of stress doing homework. Perhaps the most useful part of problem solving for the homework problem was defining the problem accurately. Through active discussion, it became clear that "homework stress" really represented a set of problems: Adele's worries about making a mistake, Adele wanting to spend less time on homework and more time with her mother, Adele not wanting to miss out on family activities, and Adele finding her brother's behavior distracting. Each problem was then addressed individually. Through the We Can Solve Problems Together module, the therapist was able to incorporate other behavioral techniques, such as having "practicing making mistakes" be one of the solutions to Adele's worries about making a mistake to encourage opportunities for exposure. Three of the problems were discussed in two separate sessions and the fourth problem was assigned to complete together at home, and then reviewed in session.

Final Phase of Treatment

This treatment phase focused on solidifying existing skills and relapse prevention. Doing fun activities together was a preexisting strength of the family, so the focus on this skill was brief, but included reinforcing the importance of maintaining these activities. Communication and problem-solving skills were furthered by continued practice. Each week the parents and Adele would report on the week's upward spirals and skills used, and raise any downward spirals to focus on in session. The therapist gradually transferred leadership of the discussion to Adele and her parents, so that they discussed the problem, identified the skill(s) to use, and used those skills with decreasing therapist input. By the final session, Adele and her parents agreed that they were ready to use these skills independently, and that downward spirals were significantly less frequent and severe compared to when they started treatment.

Case Vignette 3: Building Resilience Into the System

The case of Matthew is from "Family-Focused Treatment for Childhood Depression: Model and Case Illustrations" by M. C. Tompson, D. A. Langer, J. L. Hughes, & J. R. Asarnow, 2017, *Cognitive and Behavioral Practice*, 24(3), pp. 269–287. © 2017 by Elsevier. Reprinted with permission from Elsevier.

Initial Presentation

Matthew was an 8-year-old European-American boy in the second grade living with his parents and 18-month-old sister. He and his mother reported that his depressive symptoms began about 1 year previously. He began therapy at that point, but the therapy was disrupted when the family relocated 6 months ago due to his father's job. They moved from a small suburb with a strong family-support system to a large city with little support. Matthew reported being "mostly excited" about the move, as he liked the adventure of it, but "really sad" to be away from his friends and family. Although he had close friends at his former school, he had difficulty making friends at his new school. His depressive symptoms worsened around the time of the move. Matthew's mother described him as "very, very smart" and "articulate," with restricted interests, including dinosaurs and airplanes. She noted that although he could be interested in and engage with others in conversations about other topics, he preferred to focus on his main interests. Although early evaluation had ruled out an autism spectrum disorder, Matthew had a number of social challenges. Despite frequent dysphoria, Matthew was not anhedonic, as he reported being happy at home, feeling close to both parents, and enjoying family activities, such as camping, going to the library, and doing science experiments. Matthew's mother reported that the foursome spent a lot of time together, particularly since moving, as they did not know many local families. She reported her own history of severe depression: Having been treated successfully with medication and therapy, she reported being symptom free for the past year.

Early Phase of Treatment

Matthew and his mother attended 15 sessions of FFT-CD, and his father joined in when his work and travel schedule allowed, approximately one third of sessions. In the first few weeks, they focused on communication skills. They enjoyed the "saying what you like" skill, using the token system both in and out of session to reinforce helpful statements and behaviors. Matthew excitedly reported in Session 3, "We traded dots at home!" The presence of his younger sibling in sessions was challenging at times, as it divided his mother's attention. However, the therapist included her when possible (e.g., giving her tokens to use/drool on), and the mother made sure to have toys and snacks available to distract her. Matthew did not seem to mind having the sister in the room and even included her in certain silly examples and exercises.

Matthew expressed some frustration that his father, who worked full time, was not in the sessions. Matthew and his mother collaborated with the therapist to identify ways in which the father might be involved in treatment, including asking him to attend sessions, teaching the materials to him at dinner after sessions, and including him in weekly practice assignments. Matthew expressed interest in all of these ideas and, with obvious delight, was successful in bringing his father to session following this discussion. The father's participation in the skills review and role-plays made it clear that the family had been practicing skills at home. Matthew's father excelled at reinforcing that Matthew had taught him skills, stating "I learned about that from him" and praising his skills use in session. The family was readily able to apply the concepts to their family interactions. Matthew particularly enjoyed the silly examples in the role-plays (e.g., "I liked it when you went bowling in your pajamas"), giggling with his parents.

In a brief individual meeting, the father noted his concerns with Matthew's ability to regulate emotions, as he was easily angry and struggled to recover. The therapist provided additional psychoeducation about the role of irritability in childhood depression and how FFT-CD skills could help Matthew learn ways to manage his emotions through interactions with others. Although the emotion thermometer is often not introduced until the We Can Solve Problems Together module, it was implemented to aid Matthew in monitoring the intensity of emotions.

Middle Phase of Treatment

The next phase of treatment focused on identifying downward spirals and addressing them with communication or problem solving. Matthew's father frequently joined, and the family was active and engaged during treatment sessions. Parental marital tension became apparent, but the therapist was able to keep the family focused on role-plays and Matthew's perspectives to keep the tension from fully playing out in session. Sample downward spirals included conflict related to chores and computer time, as well as spirals related to parents' mood states and stress levels. For example, the mother was able to identify that when she has had a day where she felt more down, stressed, or not supported, she was more likely to be "short" with Matthew, which then would lead him into a downward spiral (see Figure 9). The family used the Things We Do Affect How We Feel module to focus on building more positive experiences in the family such that everyone's stress was reduced, helping to prevent some of these spirals. Additionally, the therapist met separately with the mother to check in and gave referrals for her to see a therapist due to her increased depressive symptoms. Other downward spirals related to Matthew's difficulty in developing and maintaining friendships. The family and therapist used the Things We Do Affect How We Feel module to brainstorm activities Matthew could do with friends, such as his mother setting up play dates and Matthew joining classes at the local community center, as well as setting up some summer day camps.

The therapist introduced the We Can Solve Problems Together module by highlighting the many problems Matthew had successfully solved after moving to the city, highlighting his strength in this area. The family decided to address the problem of eating dinner together, as the father had been working later and others were hungry earlier. The family brainstormed possibilities, with the therapist highlighting but not judging any possibilities and throwing in silly ideas as well (e.g., Matthew and his mother go to work and eat on the father's desk). This exercise occasionally tripped on additional marital conflict, but the therapist was able to keep the focus on the defined problem by meeting briefly with parents to explicitly acknowledge the conflict, redirect the focus of the treatment to the child, and refer the parents for couples' treatment.

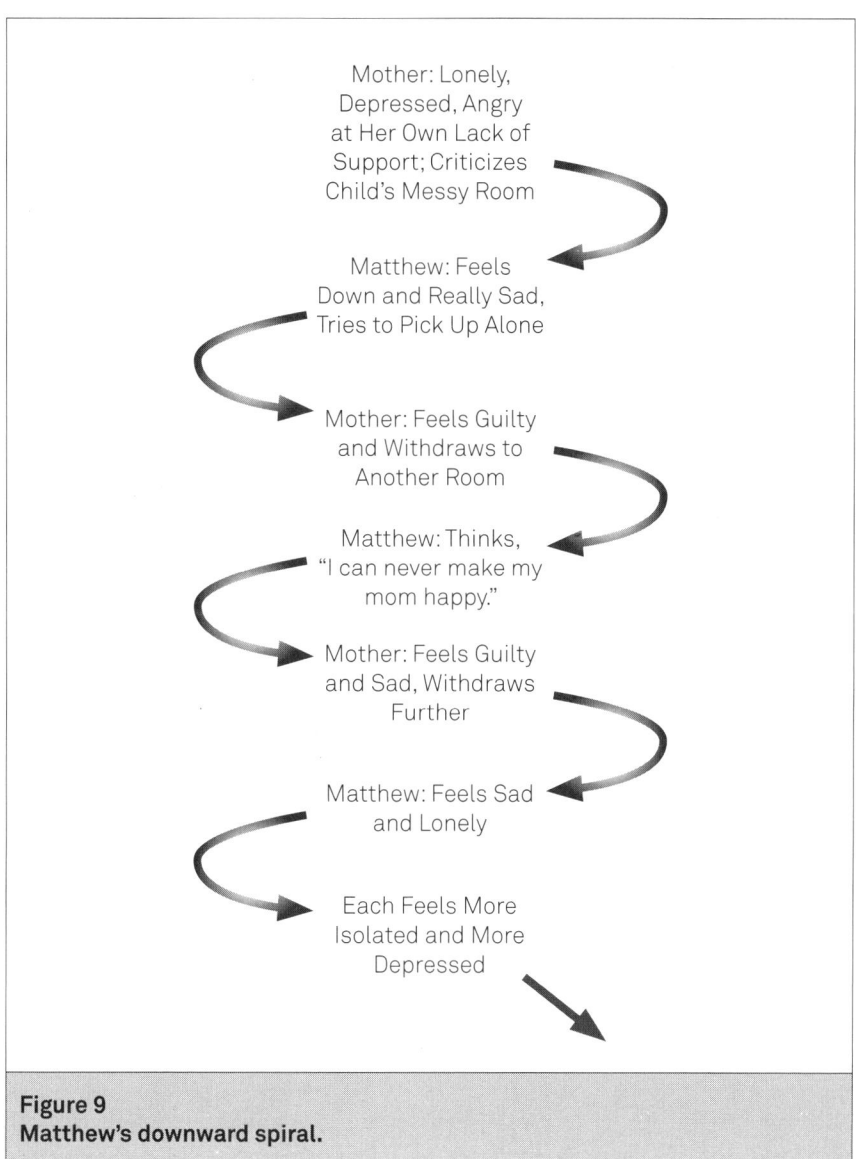

Figure 9
Matthew's downward spiral.

Final Phase of Treatment

Matthew demonstrated great gains during FFT-CD and clearly benefited from learning the skills, as evidenced by his reporting using the strategies at home. During treatment, it became increasingly apparent that his parents were struggling in their relationship. Fortunately, FFT-CD had helped to build resilience into the system such that his parents were able to use the skills to support Matthew's continued improvement, even while making some difficult decisions about their family situation. In Session 11, his mother reported that she and his father had decided to separate. Following treatment completion, one booster session was conducted at the time of the follow-up assessment. Matthew had continued to maintain gains made during the treatment.

6

Further Reading

Understanding the Nature of Depression in Youth

Bernaras, E., Jaureguizar, J., & Garaigordobil, M. (2019). Child and adolescent depression: A review of theories, evaluation instruments, prevention programs, and treatments. *Frontiers in Psychology, 10*, 543. https://doi.org/10.3389/fpsyg.2019.00543

Hankin, B. L. (2012). Future directions in vulnerability to depression among youth: Integrating risk factors and processes across multiple levels of analysis. *Journal of Clinical Child & Adolescent Psychology, 41*(5), 695–718. https://doi.org/10.1080/15374416.2012.711708

Treatment of Depression in Youth

Kennard, B. D., Hughes, J. L., & Foxwell, A. A. (2016). *CBT for depression in children and adolescents: A guide to relapse prevention*. Guilford Press.

Reynolds, W. M., & Johnston, H. F. (Eds.). (2013). *Handbook of depression in children and adolescents*. Springer Science & Business Media.

Weersing, V. R., Jeffreys, M., Do, M. C. T., Schwartz, K. T., & Bolano, C. (2017). Evidence base update of psychosocial treatments for child and adolescent depression. *Journal of Clinical Child & Adolescent Psychology, 46*(1), 11–43. https://doi.org/10.1080/15374416.2016.1220310

Family-Focused Treatment for Childhood Depression

Tompson, M. C., Boger, K. D., & Asarnow, J. R. (2012). Enhancing the developmental appropriateness of treatment for depression in youth: Integrating the family in treatment. *Child Psychiatric Clinics of North America, 21*(3), 345–384. https://doi.org/10.1016/j.chc.2012.01.003

Tompson, M. C., Langer, D. A., & Asarnow, J. R. (2020). Development and efficacy of a family-focused treatment for depression in childhood. *Journal of Affective Disorders, 276*, 686–695. https://doi.org/10.1016/j.jad.2020.06.057

Other Family Approaches for Mood Disorders in Youth

Diamond, G. S., Diamond, G. M., & Levy, S. A. (2014). *Attachment-based therapy for depressed adolescents*. American Psychological Association. https://doi.org/10.1037/14296-000

Dietz, L. J., Mufson, L., & Weinberg, R. B. (2018). *Family-based interpersonal therapy for depressed preadolescents*. Oxford University Press. https://doi.org/10.1093/med-psych/9780190640033.001.0001

Lenze, S. N., Pautsch, J., & Luby, J. (2011). Parent–child interaction therapy emotion development: A novel treatment for depression in preschool children. *Depression and Anxiety, 28*(2), 153–159. https://doi.org/10.1002/da.20770

Miklowitz, D. J., & George, E. L. (2007). *The bipolar teen: What you can do to help your child and your family*. Guilford Press.

7

References

Abela, J. R. Z., & Hankin, B. L. (2008). Cognitive vulnerability to depression in children and adolescents: A developmental psychopathology perspective. In J. R. Z. Abela & B. L. Hankin (Eds.), *Handbook of depression in children and adolescents* (pp. 35–78). Guilford Press.

Abramson, L. Y., Alloy, L. B., & Metalsky, G. I. (2013). The hopelessness theory of depression: Current status and future directions. In N. L. Stein, B. Leventhal, & T. R. Trabasso (Eds.), *Psychological and biological approaches to emotion* (pp. 351–376). Psychology Press.

Achenbach, T. M. (2013). *DSM guide for the ASEBA*. University of Vermont, Research Center for Children, Youth, & Families.

Agoston, A. M., & Rudolph, K. D. (2016). Interactive contributions of cumulative peer stress and executive function deficits to depression in early adolescence. *Journal of Early Adolescence, 36*(8), 1070–1094. https://doi.org/10.1177/0272431615593176

Alegria, M., Vallas, M., & Pumariega, A. J. (2010). Racial and ethnic disparities in pediatric mental health. *Child and Adolescent Psychiatric Clinics of North America, 19*(4), 759–774. https://doi.org/10.1016/j.chc.2010.07.001

Alloy, L. B., Abramson, L. Y., Tashman, N. A., Berrebbi, D. S., Hogan, M. E., Whitehouse, W. G., Crossfield, A. G., & Morocco, A. (2001). Developmental origins of cognitive vulnerability to depression: Parenting, cognitive, and inferential feedback styles of the parents of individuals at high and low cognitive risk for depression. *Cognitive Therapy and Research, 25*(4), 397–423. https://doi.org/10.1023/A:1005527218169

American Academy of Pediatrics. (2021, October 19). AAP, AACAP, CHA declare national emergency in children's mental health. AAP News. https://publications.aap.org/aapnews/news/17718

American Psychiatric Association. (1980). *Diagnostic and statistical manual of mental disorders* (3rd ed.).

American Psychiatric Association. (1987). *Diagnostic and statistical manual of mental disorders* (3rd ed., rev.).

American Psychiatric Association. (1994). *Diagnostic and statistical manual of mental disorders* (4th ed.).

American Psychiatric Association. (2000). *Diagnostic and statistical manual of mental disorders* (4th ed., text rev.).

American Psychiatric Association. (2013). *Diagnostic and statistical manual of mental disorders* (5th ed.).

American Psychological Association, Presidential Task Force on Evidence-Based Practice. (2006). Evidence-based practice in psychology. *American Psychologist, 61*(4), 271–285. https://doi.org/10.1037/0003-066X.61.4.271

Anderson, J. C., Williams, S., McGee, R., & Silva, P. A. (1987). DSM-III disorders in preadolescent children: Prevalence in a large sample from the general population. *Archives of General Psychiatry, 44*(1), 69–76. https://doi.org/10.1001/archpsyc.1987.01800130081010

Angold, A., & Costello, E. J. (1993). Depressive comorbidity in children and adolescents: Empirical, theoretical, and methodological issues. *Annual Progress in Child Psychiatry and Child Development, 150*(12), 441–468.

Angold, A., & Costello, J. (2000). The child and adolescent psychiatric assessment (CAPA). *Journal of the American Academy of Child & Adolescent Psychiatry, 39*(1), 39–48. https://doi.org/10.1097/00004583-200001000-00015

Angold, A., Costello, E. J., Messer, S. C., Pickles, A., Winder, F., & Silver, D. (1995). The development of a short questionnaire for use in epidemiological studies of depression in children and adolescents. *International Journal of Methods in Psychiatric Research, 5*(4), 237–249.

Angold, A., Costello, E. J., & Worthman, C. M. (1998). Puberty and depression: The roles of age, pubertal status and pubertal timing. *Psychological Medicine, 28*(1), 51–61. https://doi.org/10.1017/S003329179700593X

Angold, A., Erkanli, A., Farmer, E. M. Z., Fairbank, J. A., Burns, B. J., Keeler, G., & Costello, E. J. (2002). Psychiatric disorder, impairment, and service use in rural African American and White youth. *Archives of General Psychiatry, 59*(10), 893–904. https://doi.org/10.1001/archpsyc.59.10.893

Asarnow, J. R., & Carlson, G. A. (1985). Depression self-rating scale: Utility with child psychiatric inpatients. *Journal of Consulting and Clinical Psychology, 53*(4), 491–499. https://doi.org/10.1037/0022-006X.53.4.491

Asarnow, J. R., Jaycox, L. H., Duan, N., LaBorde, A. P., Rea, M. M., Murray, P., Anderson, M., Landon, C., Tang, L., & Wells, K. B. (2005). Effectiveness of a quality improvement intervention for adolescent depression in primary care clinics: A randomized controlled trial. *JAMA: Journal of the American Medical Association, 293*(3), 311–319. https://doi.org/10.1001/jama.293.3.311

Asarnow, J. R., Tompson, M. C., Klomhaus, A. M., Babeva, K., Langer, D. A., & Sugar, C. A. (2020). Randomized controlled trial of family-focused treatment for child depression compared to individual psychotherapy: One-year outcomes. *Journal of Child Psychology and Psychiatry, and Allied Disciplines, 61*(6), 662–671. https://doi.org/10.1111/jcpp.13162

Avenevoli, S., & Merikangas, K. (2006). Implications of high-risk family studies for prevention of depression. *American Journal of Preventive Medicine, 31*(Suppl. 1), S126–S135. https://doi.org/10.1016/j.amepre.2006.07.003

Baldwin, M. W. (1992). Relational schemas and the processing of social information. *Psychological Bulletin, 112*(3), 461–484. https://doi.org/10.1037/0033-2909.112.3.461

Beck, A. T., & Bredemeier, K. (2016). A unified model of depression: Integrating clinical, cognitive, biological, and evolutionary perspectives. *Clinical Psychological Science, 4*(4), 596–619. https://doi.org/10.1177/2167702616628523

Beck, A. T., Steer, G. K., & Brown, G. K. (1996). *Beck depression inventory: Manual* (2nd ed.). Psychological Corporation.

Bennett, D. S. (1994). Depression among children with chronic medical problems: A meta-analysis. *Journal of Pediatric Psychology, 19*(2), 149–169. https://doi.org/10.1093/jpepsy/19.2.149

Bernaras, E., Jaureguizar, J., & Garaigordobil, M. (2019). Child and adolescent depression: A review of theories, evaluation instruments, prevention programs, and treatments. *Frontiers in Psychology, 10*, 543. https://doi.org/10.3389/fpsyg.2019.00543

Bird, H. R., Gould, M. S., & Staghezza, B. M. (1993). Patterns of diagnostic comorbidity in a community sample of children aged 9 through 16 years. *Journal of the American Academy of Child & Adolescent Psychiatry, 32*(2), 361–368. https://doi.org/10.1097/00004583-199303000-00018

Birmaher, B., Brent, D., AACAP Work Group on Quality Issues, Bernet, W., Bukstein, O., Walter, H., Benson, R. S., Chrisman, A., Farchione, T., Greenhill, L., Hamilton, J., Keable, H., Kinlan, J., Schoetle, U., Stock, S., Ptakowski, K. K., & Medicus, J. (2007). Practice parameter for the assessment and treatment of children and adolescents with depressive disorders. *Journal of the American Academy of Child & Adolescent Psychiatry, 46*(11), 1503–1526. https://doi.org/10.1097/chi.0b013e318145ae1c

Birmaher, B., Ryan, N. D., Williamson, D. E., Brent, D. A., Kaufman, J., Dahl, R. E., Perel, J., & Nelson, B. (1996). Childhood and adolescent depression: A review of the past 10 years. Part I. *Journal of the American Academy of Child & Adolescent*

Psychiatry, 35(12), 1427–1439. https://doi.org/10.1097/00004583-199612000-00008

Birmaher, B., Williamson, D. E., Dahl, R. E., Axelson, D. A., Kaufman, J., Dorn, L. D., & Ryan, N. D. (2004). Clinical presentation and course of depression in youth: Does onset in childhood differ from onset in adolescence? *Journal of the American Academy of Child & Adolescent Psychiatry, 43*(1), 63–70. https://doi.org/10.1097/00004583-200401000-00015

Blue Cross Blue Shield. (2018, May 10). *Major depression: The impact on overall health.* https://www.bcbs.com/the-health-of-america/reports/major-depression-the-impact-overall-health

Burkhouse, K. L., Uhrlass, D. J., Stone, L. B., Knopik, V. S., & Gibb, B. E. (2012). Expressed emotion-criticism and risk of depression onset in children. *Journal of Clinical Child & Adolescent Psychology, 41*(6), 771–777. https://doi.org/10.1080/15374416.2012.703122

Canino, G., Shrout, P. E., Rubio-Stipec, M., Bird, H. R., Bravo, M., Ramirez, R., Chavez, L., Alegria, M., Bauermeister, J. J., Hohmann, A., Ribera, J., Garcia, P., & Martinez-Taboas, A. (2004). The DSM-IV rates of child and adolescent disorders in Puerto Rico: Prevalence, correlates, service use, and the effects of impairment. *Archives of General Psychiatry, 61*(1), 85–93. https://doi.org/10.1001/archpsyc.61.1.85

Cao, J., Truong, A. L., Banu, S., Shah, A. A., Sabharwal, A., & Moukaddam, N. (2020). Tracking and predicting depressive symptoms of adolescents using smartphone-based self-reports, parental evaluations, and passive phone sensor data: Development and usability study. *JMIR Mental Health, 7*(1), e14045. https://doi.org/10.2196/14045

Cappelli, M., Gray, C., Zemek, R., Cloutier, P., Kennedy, A., Glennie, E., Doucet, G., & Lyons, J. S. (2012). The HEADS-ED: A rapid mental health screening tool for pediatric patients in the emergency department. *Pediatrics, 130*(2), e321–327. https://doi.org/10.1542/peds.2011-3798

Carlson, G. A., & Cantwell, D. P. (1980). Unmasking masked depression in children and adolescents. *American Journal of Psychiatry, 137*(4), 445–449. https://doi.org/10.1176/ajp.137.4.445

Cash, S. J., & Bridge, J. A. (2009). Epidemiology of youth suicide and suicidal behavior. *Current Opinion in Pediatrics, 21*(5), 613–619. https://doi.org/10.1097/MOP.0b013e32833063e1

Chambless, D. L., & Hollon, S. D. (1998). Defining empirically supported therapies. *Journal of Consulting and Clinical Psychology, 66*(1), 7–18. https://doi.org/10.1037/0022-006X.66.1.7

Cipriani, A., Zhou, X., Del Giovane, C., Hetrick, S. E., Qin, B., Whittington, C., Coghill, D., Zhang, Y., Hazell, P., Leucht, S., Cuijpers, P., Pu, J., Cohen, D., Ravindran, A. B., Liu, Y., Michael, K. D., Yang, L., Liu, L., & Xie, P. (2016). Comparative efficacy and tolerability of antidepressants for major depressive disorder in children and adolescents: A network meta-analysis. *The Lancet, 388*(10047), 881–890. https://doi.org/10.1016/S0140-6736(16)30385-3

Clark, L. A., & Watson, D. (1991). Tripartite model of anxiety and depression: Psychometric evidence and taxonomic implications. *Journal of Abnormal Psychology, 100*(3), 316–336. https://doi.org/10.1037/0021-843X.100.3.316

Cohen, J. A., & Mannarino, A. P. (1996). A treatment outcome study for sexually abused preschool children: Initial findings. *Journal of the American Academy of Child & Adolescent Psychiatry, 35*(1), 42–50. https://doi.org/10.1097/00004583-199601000-00011

Cole, D. A., & Turner, J. E., Jr. (1993). Models of cognitive mediation and moderation in child depression. *Journal of Abnormal Psychology, 102*(2), 271–281. https://doi.org/10.1037/0021-843X.102.2.271

Conley, C. S., & Rudolph, K. D. (2009). The emerging sex difference in adolescent depression: Interacting contributions of puberty and peer stress. *Development and Psychopathology, 21*(2), 593–620. https://doi.org/10.1017/S0954579409000327

Costello, E. J., Mustillo, S., Erkanli, A., Keeler, G., & Angold, A. (2003). Prevalence and development of psychiatric disorders in childhood and adolescence. *Archives of General Psychiatry, 60*(8), 837–844. https://doi.org/10.1001/archpsyc.60.8.837

De Los Reyes, A., Goodman, K. L., Kliewer, W., & Reid-Quiñones, K. (2008). Whose depression relates to discrepancies? Testing relations between informant characteristics and informant discrepancies from both informants' perspectives. *Psychological Assessment, 20*(2), 139–149.

De Los Reyes, A., & Kazdin, A. E. (2005). Informant discrepancies in the assessment of childhood psychopathology: A critical review, theoretical framework, and recommendations for further study. *Psychological Bulletin, 131*(4), 483–509. https://doi.org/10.1037/0033-2909.131.4.483

Dietz, L. J., Weinberg, R. J., Brent, D. A., & Mufson, L. (2015). Family-based interpersonal psychotherapy for depressed preadolescents: Examining efficacy and potential treatment mechanisms. *Journal of the American Academy of Child & Adolescent Psychiatry, 54*(3), 191–199. https://doi.org/10.1016/j.jaac.2014.12.011

Devlin, N. J., & Brooks, R. (2017). EQ-5D and the EuroQol Group: Past, present and future. *Applied Health Economics and Health Policy, 15*(2), 127–137. https://doi.org/10.1007/s40258-017-0310-5

Fassett-Carman, A., Hankin, B. L., & Snyder, H. R. (2019). Appraisals of dependent stressor controllability and severity are associated with depression and anxiety symptoms in youth. *Anxiety, Stress & Coping, 32*(1), 32–49. https://doi.org/10.1080/10615806.2018.1532504

Federal Interagency Forum on Child and Family Statistics. (2023). *America's children in brief: Key national indicators of well-being, 2023.* https://www.childstats.gov/pdf/ac2023/ac_23.pdf

Friedman, R. A. (2014). Antidepressants' black-box warning: 10 years later. *New England Journal of Medicine, 371*(18), 1666–1668. https://doi.org/10.1056/NEJMp1408480

Frost, L. A., Moffitt, T. E., & McGee, R. (1989). Neuropsychological correlates of psychopathology in an unselected cohort of young adolescents. *Journal of Abnormal Psychology, 98*(3), 307–313. https://doi.org/10.1037/0021-843X.98.3.307

Garber, J., Clarke, G. N., Weersing, V. R., Beardslee, W. R., Brent, D. A., Gladstone, T. R., DeBar, L. L., Lynch, F. L., D'Angelo, E., Hollon, S. D., Shamseddeen, W., & Iyengar, S. (2009). Prevention of depression in at-risk adolescents: A randomized controlled trial. *JAMA, 301*(21), 2215–2224. https://doi.org/10.1001/jama.2009.788

Garber, J., & Flynn, C. (2001). Vulnerability to depression in childhood and adolescence. In R. E. Ingram & J. M. Price (Eds.), *Vulnerability to psychopathology: Risk across the lifespan* (pp. 175–225). Guilford Press.

Garber, J., & Martin, N. C. (2002). Negative cognitions in offspring of depressed parents: Mechanisms of risk. In S. H. Goodman & I. H. Gotlib (Eds.), *Children of depressed parents: Mechanisms of risk and implications for treatment* (pp. 121–153). American Psychological Association.

Gee, D. G., Gabard-Durnam, L., Telzer, E. H., Humphreys, K. L., Goff, B., Shapiro, M., Flannery, J., Lumian, D. S., Fareri, D. S., Caldera, C., & Tottenham, N. (2014). Maternal buffering of human amygdala-prefrontal circuitry during childhood but not during adolescence. *Psychological Science, 25*(11), 2067–2078. https://doi.org/10.1177/0956797614550878

Gershon, E., Hamovit, J., Guroff, J. J., Dibble, E., Leckman, J. F., Sceery, W., Targum, S. D., Nurnberger, J. I., Jr., Goldin, L. R., & Bunney, W. E., Jr. (1982). A family study of schizoaffective bipolar I, bipolar II, unipolar, and normal control probands. *Archives of General Psychiatry, 39*(10), 1157–1167. https://doi.org/10.1001/archpsyc.1982.04290100031006

Goodman, S. H., & Gotlib, I. H. (1999). Risk for psychopathology in the children of depressed mothers: A developmental model for understanding mechanisms of transmission. *Psychological Review, 106*(3), 458–490. https://doi.org/10.1037/0033-295X.106.3.458

Goodman, S. H., Rouse, M. H., Connell, A. M., Broth, M. R., Hall, C. M., & Heyward, D. (2011). Maternal depression and child psychopathology: A meta-analytic review. *Clinical Child and Family Psychology Review, 14*(1), 1–27. https://doi.org/10.1007/s10567-010-0080-1

Greene, R. W., & Ablon, J. S. (2005). *Treating explosive kids: The collaborative problem-solving approach*. Guilford Press.

Guz, S., Kattari, S. K., Atteberry-Ash, B., Klemmer, C. L., Call, J., & Kattari, L. (2021). Depression and suicide risk at the cross-section of sexual orientation and gender identity for youth. *Journal of Adolescent Health, 68*(2), 317–323. https://doi.org/10.1016/j.jadohealth.2020.06.008

Hammen, C. (2006). Stress generation in depression: Reflections on origins, research, and future directions. *Journal of Clinical Psychology, 62*(9), 1065–1082. https://doi.org/10.1002/jclp.20293

Hammen, C. C., Hazel, N. A., Brennan, P. A., & Najman, J. J. (2012). Intergenerational transmission and continuity of stress and depression: Depressed women and their offspring in 20 years of follow-up. *Psychological Medicine, 42*(5), 931–942. https://doi.org/10.1017/S0033291711001978

Hankin, B. L. (2012). Future directions in vulnerability to depression among youth: Integrating risk factors and processes across multiple levels of analysis. *Journal of Clinical Child & Adolescent Psychology, 41*(5), 695–718. https://doi.org/10.1080/15374416.2012.711708

Hankin, B. L., Abramson, L. Y., Moffitt, T. E., Silva, P. A., McGee, R., & Angell, K. E. (1998). Development of depression from preadolescence to young adulthood: Emerging gender differences in a 10-year longitudinal study. *Journal of Abnormal Psychology, 107*(1), 128–140. https://doi.org/10.1037/0021-843X.107.1.128

Hazel, N. A., Oppenheimer, C. W., Technow, J. R., Young, J. F., & Hankin, B. L. (2014). Parent relationship quality buffers against the effect of peer stressors on depressive symptoms from middle childhood to adolescence. *Developmental Psychology, 50*(8), 2115–2123. https://doi.org/10.1037/a0037192

Ingram, R. E., & Luxton, D. D. (2005). Vulnerability-stress models. In B. L. Hankin & J. R. Z. Abela (Eds.), *Development of psychopathology: A vulnerability stress perspective* (pp. 32–46). Sage Publications. https://doi.org/10.435/978/452231655.n2

Ivarsson, T., Lidberg, A., & Gillberg, C. (1994). The Birleson Depression Self-Rating Scale (DSRS): Clinical evaluation in an adolescent inpatient population. *Journal of Affective Disorders, 32*(2), 115–125. https://doi.org/10.1016/0165-0327(94)90069-8

Jaffee, S. R., Moffitt, T. E., Caspi, A., Fombonne, E., Poulton, R., & Martin, J. (2002). Differences in early childhood risk factors for juvenile-onset and adult-onset depression. *Archives of General Psychiatry, 59*(3), 215–222. https://doi.org/10.1001/archpsyc.59.3.215

Johnson, K. C., LeBlanc, A. J., Sterzing, P. R., Deardorff, J., Antin, T., & Bockting, W. O. (2020). Trans adolescents' perceptions and experiences of their parents' supportive and rejecting behaviors. *Journal of Counseling Psychology, 67*(2), 156. https://doi.org/10.1037/cou0000419

Joiner, T., & Coyne, J. C. (Eds.). (1999). *The interactional nature of depression: Advances in interpersonal approaches*. American Psychological Association. https://doi.org/10.1037/10311-000

Kashani, J. H., Carlson, G. A., Beck, N. C., Hoeper, E. W., Corcoran, C. M., McAllister, J. A., Fallahi, C., Rosenberg, T. K., & Reid, J. C. (1987). Depression, depressive symptoms, and depressed mood among a community sample of adolescents. *American Journal of Psychiatry, 144*(7), 931–934. https://doi.org/10.1176/ajp.144.7.931

Kashani, J. H., Holcomb, W. R., & Orvaschel, H. (1986). Depression and depressive symptoms in preschool children from the general population. *American Journal of Psychiatry, 143*(9), 1138–1143. https://doi.org/10.1176/ajp.143.9.1138

Kashani, J. H., McGee, R. O., Clarkson, S. E., Anderson, J. C., Walton, L. A., Williams, S., Silva, P. A., Robins, A. J., Cytryn, L., & McKnew, D. H. (1983). Depression in a sample of 9-year-old children: Prevalence and associated characteristics. *Archives of General Psychiatry, 40*(11), 1217-1223. https://doi.org/10.1001/archpsyc.1983.01790100063009

Kaufman, J., Birmaher, B., Brent, D., Rao, U., Flynn, C., Moreci, P., Williamson, D., & Ryan, N. (1997). Schedule for Affective Disorders and Schizophrenia for School-Age Children-Present and Lifetime Version (K-SADS-PL): Initial reliability and validity data. *Journal of the American Academy of Child & Adolescent Psychiatry, 36*(7), 980-988. https://doi.org/10.1097/00004583-199707000-00021

Kendler, K. S., & Prescott, C. A. (1999). A population-based twin study of lifetime major depression in men and women. *Archives of General Psychiatry, 56*(1), 39-44. https://doi.org/10.1001/archpsyc.56.1.39

Kerestes, R., Davey, C. G., Stephanou, K., Whittle, S., & Harrison, B. J. (2013). Functional brain imaging studies of youth depression: A systematic review. *NeuroImage Clinical, 4*, 209-231. https://doi.org/10.1016/j.nicl.2013.11.009

Kessler, R. C., & Üstün, T. B. (2004). The World Mental Health (WMH) Survey Initiative version of the World Health Organization (WHO) Composite International Diagnostic Interview (CIDI). *International Journal of Methods in Psychiatric Research, 13*(2), 93-121. https://doi.org/10.1002/mpr.168

Kinyanda, E., Weiss, H. A., Mungherera, M., Onyango-Mangen, P., Ngabirano, E., Kajungu, R., Kagugube, J., Muhwezi, W., Muron, J., & Patel, V. (2013). Prevalence and risk factors of attempted suicide in adult war-affected population of eastern Uganda. *Crisis, 34*(5), 314-323. https://doi.org/10.1027/0227-5910/a000196

Klein, D. N., Kotov, R., & Bufferd, S. J. (2011). Personality and depression: Explanatory models and review of the evidence. *Annual Review of Clinical Psychology, 7*, 269-295. https://doi.org/10.1146/annurev-clinpsy-032210-104540

Klomek, A. B., Marrocco, F., Kleinman, M., Schonfeld, I. S., & Gould, M. S. (2007). Bullying, depression, and suicidality in adolescents. *Journal of the American Academy of Child & Adolescent Psychiatry, 46*(1), 40-49. https://doi.org/10.1097/01.chi.0000242237.84925.18

Kovacs, M. (1996). The course of childhood-onset depressive disorders. *Psychiatric Annals, 26*(6), 326-330. https://doi.org/10.3928/0048-5713-19960601-10

Kovacs, M. (2011). *The Children's Depression Inventory (CDI-2)*. Pearson Education.

Kovacs, M., Akiskal, H. S., Gatsonis, C., & Parrone, P. L. (1994). Childhood-onset dysthymic disorder: Clinical features and prospective naturalistic outcome. *Archives of General Psychiatry, 51*(5), 365-374. https://doi.org/10.1001/archpsyc.1994.03950050025003

Kovacs, M., Devlin, B., Pollock, M., Richards, C., & Mukerji, P. (1997). A controlled family history study of childhood-onset depressive disorder. *Archives of General Psychiatry, 54*(7), 613-623. https://doi.org/10.1001/archpsyc.1997.01830190033004

Kovacs, M., Feinberg, T. L., Crouse-Novak, M. A., Paulauskas, S. L., & Finkelstein, R. (1984a). Depressive disorders in childhood: I. A longitudinal prospective study of characteristics and recovery. *Archives of General Psychiatry, 41*(3), 229-237. https://doi.org/10.1001/archpsyc.1984.01790140019002

Kovacs, M., Feinberg, T. L., Crouse-Novak, M., Paulauskas, S. L., Pollock, M., & Finkelstein, R. (1984b). Depressive disorders in childhood: II. A longitudinal study of the risk for a subsequent major depression. *Archives of General Psychiatry, 41*(7), 643-649. https://doi.org/10.1001/archpsyc.1984.01790140019002

Kovacs, M., Obrosky, S., & George, C. (2016). The course of major depressive disorder from childhood to young adulthood: Recovery and recurrence in a longitudinal observational study. *Journal of Affective Disorders, 203*, 374-381. https://doi.org/10.1016/j.jad.2016.05.042

Kowalski, R. M., & Limber, S. P. (2013). Psychological, physical, and academic correlates of cyberbullying and traditional bullying. *Journal of Adolescent Health, 53*(1, Suppl.), S13-S20. https://doi.org/10.1016/j.jadohealth.2012.09.018

Kroenke, K., Spitzer, R. L., & Williams, J. B. W. (2001). The PHQ-9: Validity of a brief depression severity measure. *Journal of General Internal Medicine, 16*(3), 606-613. https://doi.org/10.1046/j.1525-1497.2001.016009606.x

Kroenke, K., Spitzer, R. L., & Williams, J. B. W. (2003). Patient Health Questionnaire-2: Validity of a two-item depression screener. *Medical Care, 41*(11), 1284-1292. https://doi.org/10.1097/01.MLR.0000093487.78664.3C

Lachar, D., Randle, S. L., Harper, R. A., Scott-Gurnell, K. C., Lewis, K. R., Santos, C. W., Saunders, A. E., Pearson, D. A., Loveland, K. A., & Morgan, S. T. (2001). The brief psychiatric rating scale for children (BPRS-C): Validity and reliability of an anchored version. *Journal of the American Academy of Child & Adolescent Psychiatry, 40*(3), 333-340. https://doi.org/10.1097/00004583-200103000-00013

Ladd, G. W., & Troop-Gordon, W. (2003). The role of chronic peer difficulties in the development of children's psychological adjustment problems. *Child Development, 74*(5), 1344-1367. https://doi.org/10.1111/1467-8624.00611

Langer, D. A., Holly, L. E., Wills, C. E., Tompson, M. C., & Chorpita, B. F. (2022). Shared decision-making for youth psychotherapy: A preliminary randomized clinical trial on facilitating personalized treatment. *Journal of Consulting and Clinical Psychology, 90*(1), 29-38. https://doi.org/10.1037/ccp0000702

Larson, R., & Sheeber, L. (2008). The daily emotional experience of adolescents: Are adolescents more emotional, why, and how is that related to depression? In N. Allen & L. Sheeber (Eds.), *Adolescent emotional development and the emergence of depressive disorders* (pp. 11-32). Cambridge University Press.

Larzelere, R., Andersen, J., Ringle, J., & Jorgensen, D. (2004). The Child Suicide Risk Assessment: A screening measure of suicide risk in pre-adolescents. *Death Studies, 28*(9), 809-827. https://doi.org/10.1080/07481180490490861

Lay-Yee, R., Milne, B. J., Shackleton, N., Chang, K., & Davis, P. (2018). Preventing youth depression: Simulating the impact of parenting interventions. *Advances in Life Course Research, 37*(2), 15-22. https://doi.org/10.1016/j.alcr.2018.05.001

LeBlanc, J. C., Almudevar, A., Brooks, S. J., & Kutcher, S. (2002). Screening for adolescent depression: Comparison of the Kutcher Adolescent Depression Scale with the Beck Depression Inventory. *Journal of Child and Adolescent Psychopharmacology, 12*(2), 113-126. https://doi.org/10.1089/104454602760219153

Lee, K. H., Siegle, G. J., Dahl, R. E., Hooley, J. M., & Silk, J. S. (2015). Neural responses to maternal criticism in healthy youth. *Social Cognitive and Affective Neuroscience, 10*(7), 902-912. https://doi.org/10.1093/scan/nsu133

Lenze, S. N., Pautsch, J., & Luby, J. (2011). Parent-child interaction therapy emotion development: A novel treatment for depression in preschool children. *Depression and Anxiety, 28*(2), 153-159. https://doi.org/10.1002/da.20770

Lewinsohn, P. M., Hops, H., Roberts, R. E., Seeley, J. R., & Andrews, J. A. (1993). Adolescent psychopathology: I. Prevalence and incidence of depression and other DSM-III-R disorders in high school students. *Journal of Abnormal Psychology, 102*(1), 133-144. https://doi.org/10.1037/0021-843X.102.4.517

Lewis, G., Collishaw, S., Thapar, A., & Harold, G. T. (2014). Parent-child hostility and child and adolescent depression symptoms: The direction of effects, role of genetic factors and gender. *European Child & Adolescent Psychiatry, 23*(5), 317-327. https://doi.org/10.1007/s00787-013-0460-4

Lewis-Fernández, R., Aggarwal, N. K., & Kirmayer, L. J. (2020). The cultural formulation interview: Progress to date and future directions. *Transcultural Psychiatry, 57*(4), 487-496. https://doi.org/10.1177/1363461520938273

Liu, R. T., & Alloy, L. B. (2010). Stress generation in depression: A systematic review of the empirical literature and recommendations for future study. *Clinical Psychology Review, 30*(5), 582-593. https://doi.org/10.1016/j.cpr.2010.04.010

Livingston, R., Nugent, H., Rader, L., & Smith, G. (1985). Family histories of depressed and severely anxious children. *American Journal of Psychiatry, 142*(12), 1497-1499. https://doi.org/10.1176/ajp.142.12.1497

Lopez-Duran, N. L., Kovacs, M., & George, C. J. (2009). Hypothalamic-pituitary-adrenal axis dysregulation in depressed children and adolescents: A meta-analysis. *Psychoneuroendocrinology, 34*(9), 1272-1283. https://doi.org/10.1016/j.psyneuen.2009.03.016

Lovibond, S. H., & Lovibond, P. F. (1995). *Manual for the depression anxiety stress scales* (2nd ed.). Psychology Foundation.

Lu, W. (2019). Adolescent depression: National trends, risk factors, and healthcare disparities. *American Journal of Health Behavior, 43*(1), 181–194. https://doi.org/10.5993/ajhb.43.1.15

Luby, J. L., Barch, D. M., Whalen, D., Tillman, R., & Freedland, K. E. (2018). A randomized controlled trial of parent–child psychotherapy targeting emotion development for early childhood depression. *American Journal of Psychiatry, 175*(11), 1102–1110. https://doi.org/10.1176/appi.ajp.2018.18030321

Luby, J., Lenze, S., & Tillman, R. (2012). A novel early intervention for preschool depression: Findings from a pilot randomized controlled trial. *Journal of Child Psychology and Psychiatry, 53*(3), 313–322. https://doi.org/10.1111/j.1469-7610.2011.02483.x

Mahler, M. S. (1961). On sadness and grief in infancy and childhood. *Psychoanalytic Study of Childhood, 16*(1), 332–354. https://doi.org/10.1080/00797308.1961.11823214

Manos, R. C., Kanter, J. W., & Luo, W. (2011). The behavioral activation for depression scale – short form: Development and validation. *Behavior Therapy, 42*(4), 726–739. https://doi.org/10.1016/j.beth.2011.04.004

McCauley, E., Myers, K., Mitchell, J., Calderon, R., Schloredt, K., & Treder, R. (1993). Depression in young people: Initial presentation and clinical course. *Journal of the American Academy of Child & Adolescent Psychiatry, 32*(4), 714–722. https://doi.org/10.1097/00004583-199307000-00003

McGee, R., Feehan, M., Williams, S., Partridge, R., Silva, P. A., & Kelly, J. (1990). DSM-III disorders in a large sample of adolescents. *Journal of the American Academy of Child & Adolescent Psychiatry, 29*(4), 611–619. https://doi.org/10.1097/00004583-199007000-00016

McLaughlin, K. A., Hilt, L. M., & Nolen-Hoeksema, S. (2007). Racial/ethnic differences in internalizing and externalizing symptoms in adolescents. *Journal of Abnormal Child Psychology, 35*(5), 801–816. https://doi.org/10.1007/s10802-007-9128-1

Mercado, M. C., Holland, K., Leemis, R. W., Stone, D. M., & Wang, J. (2017). Trends in emergency department visits for nonfatal self-inflicted injuries among youth aged 10 to 24 years in the United States, 2001–2015. *JAMA, 318*(24), 1931–1933. https://doi.org/10.1001/jama.2017.13317

Merikangas, K. R., Cui, L., Heaton, L., Nakamura, E., Roca, C., Ding, J., Qin, H., Guo, W., Shugart, Y. Y., Zarate, C., & Angst, J. (2014). Independence of familial transmission of mania and depression: Results of the NIMH family study of affective spectrum disorders. *Molecular Psychiatry, 19*(2), 214–219. https://doi.org/10.1038/mp.2013.181

Mezulis, A. H., Hyde, J. S., & Abramson, L. Y. (2006). The developmental origins of cognitive vulnerability to depression: Temperament, parenting, and negative life events in childhood as contributors to negative cognitive style. *Developmental Psychology, 42*(6), 1012–1025. https://doi.org/10.1037/0012-1649.42.6.1012

Miklowitz, D. J., Axelson, D. A., Birmaher, B., George, E. L., Taylor, D. O., Schneck, C., Beresford, C. A., Dickinson, L. M., Craighead, W. E., & Brent, D. A. (2008). Family-focused treatment for adolescents with bipolar disorder: Results of a 2-year randomized trial. *Archives of General Psychiatry, 65*(9), 1053–1061. https://doi.org/10.1001/archpsyc.65.9.1053

Miklowitz, D. J., Biuckians, A., & Richards, J. A. (2006). Early-onset bipolar disorder: A family treatment perspective. *Development and Psychopathology, 18*(4), 1247–1265. https://doi.org/10.1017/S0954579406060603

Miklowitz, D. J., George, E. L., Richards, J. A., Simoneau, T. L., & Suddath, R. L. (2003). A randomized study of family-focused psychoeducation and pharmacotherapy in the outpatient management of bipolar disorder. *Archives of General Psychiatry, 60*(9), 904–912. https://doi.org/10.1001/archpsyc.60.9.904

Miklowitz, D. J., Schneck, C. D., George, E. L., Taylor, D. O., Sugar, C. A., Birmaher, B., Kowatch, R. A., DelBello, M., & Axelson, D. A. (2014). Pharmacotherapy and family-focused treatment for adolescents with bipolar I and II disorders: A 2-year randomized trial. *American Journal of Psychiatry, 171*(6), 658–667. https://doi.org/10.1176/appi.ajp.2014.13081130

Miranda-Mendizabal, A., Castellví, P., Parés-Badell, O., Alayo, I., Alemenara, J., Alonso, I. Blasco, M. J., Cebrià, A., Gabilondo, A., Gili, M., Lagares, C., Piqueras, J. A., Rodríguez-Jiménez, T., Rodríguez-Marín, J., Roca, M., Soto-Sanz, V., Vilagut, G., & Alonso, J. (2019). Gender differences in suicidal behavior in adolescents and young adults: Systematic review and meta-analysis of longitudinal studies. *International Journal of Public Health, 64*(2), 265–283.

Mohammadi, M. R., Alavi, S. S., Ahmadi, N., Khaleghi, A., Kamali, K., Ahmadi, A., Khaleghi, A., Kamali, K., Ahmadi, A., Hooshyari, Z., Mohamadian, F., Jaberghaderi, N., Nazaribadie, M., Sajedi, Z., Fashidfar, Z., Kaviani, N., Davasazirani, R., Shahbakhsh, A. J., Rad, M. R., ... Ashoori, S. (2019). The prevalence, comorbidity and socio-demographic factors of depressive disorder among Iranian children and adolescents: To identify the main predictors of depression. *Journal of Affective Disorders, 247*(1), 1–10. https://doi.org/10.1016/j.jad.2019.01.005

National Institute of Mental Health. (2020, October 29). *Using mobile technology to improve care for teens with depression*. https://www.nimh.nih.gov/news/research-highlights/2020/using-mobile-technology-to-improve-care-for-teens-with-depression.shtml

National Institute of Mental Health. (2022, June). *Suicide*. https://www.nih.gov/news-events/news-releases/depression-high-among-youth-victims-school-cyber-bullying-nih-researchers-report

National Institutes of Health (2010, September 12). *Depression high among youth victims of school cyber bullying, NIH researchers report: Finding underscores need to monitor, obtain treatment for recipients of cyber bulling*. News Release. https://www.nih.gov/news-events/news-releases/depression-high-among-youth-victims-school-cyber-bullying-nih-researchers-report

Ogles, B. (2009, December). *The scales*. Ohio Scales for Youth. https://sites.google.com/site/ohioscales/the-scales

Olsson, G. I., & Knorring, A. L. von (1999). Adolescent depression: Prevalence in Swedish high-school students. *Acta Psychiatrica Scandinavica, 99*(5), 324–331. https://doi.org/10.1111/j.1600-0447.1999.tb07237.x

Ormel, J., Oldehinkel, A. J., & Brilman, E. I. (2001). The interplay and etiological continuity of neuroticism, difficulties, and life events in the etiology of major and subsyndromal, first and recurrent depressive episodes in later life. *American Journal of Psychiatry, 158*(6), 885–891. https://doi.org/10.1176/appi.ajp.158.6.885

Peris, T. S., & Miklowitz, D. J. (2015). Parental expressed emotion and youth psychopathology: New directions for an old construct. *Child Psychiatry and Human Development, 46*(6), 863–873. https://doi.org/10.1007/s10578-014-0526-7

Pettit, J. W., Buitron, V., & Green, K. L. (2018). Assessment and management of suicide risk in children and adolescents. *Cognitive and Behavioral Practice, 25*(4), 460–472. https://doi.org/10.1016/j.cbpra.2018.04.001

Pfeffer, C. R., Jiang, H., & Kakuma, T. (2000). Child–Adolescent Suicidal Potential Index (CASPI): A screen for risk for early onset suicidal behavior. *Psychological Assessment, 12*(3), 304–318. https://doi.org/10.1037/1040-3590.12.3.304

Posner, K., Brown, G. K., Stanley, B., Brent, D. A., Yershova, K. V., Oquendo, M. A., Currier, G. W., Melvin, G. A., Greenhill, L., Shen, S., & Mann, J. J. (2011). The Columbia-Suicide Severity Rating Scale: Initial validity and internal consistency findings from three multisite studies with adolescents and adults. *American Journal of Psychiatry, 168*(12), 1266–1277. https://doi.org/10.1176/appi.ajp.2011.10111704

Poznanski, E. O., & Mokros, H. B. (1996). *Children's Depression Rating Scale, Revised (CDRS-R)*. WPS.

Puig-Antich, J., Goetz, D., Davies, M., Kaplan, T., Davies, S., Ostrow, L., Asnis, L., Twomey, J., Iyengar, S., & Ryan, N. D. (1989). A controlled family history study of prepubertal major depressive disorder. *Archives of General Psychiatry, 46*(5), 406-418. https://doi.org/10.1001/archpsyc.1989.01810050020005

Puig-Antich, J., Lukens, E., Davies, M., Goetz, D., Brennan-Quattrock, J., & Todak, G. (1985a). Psychosocial functioning in prepubertal major depressive disorders: I. Interpersonal relationships after sustained recovery from affective episode. *Archives of General Psychiatry, 42*(5), 500-507. https://doi.org/10.1001/archpsyc.1985.01790280093010

Puig-Antich, J., Lukens, E., Davies, M., Goetz, D., Brennan-Quattrock, J., & Todak, G. (1985b). Psychosocial functioning in prepubertal major depressive disorders: II. Interpersonal relationships after sustained recovery from affective episode. *Archives of General Psychiatry, 42*(5), 511-517. https://doi.org/10.1001/archpsyc.1985.01790280093010

Racine, N., McArthur, B. A., Cooke, J. E., Eirich, R., Zhu, J., & Madigan, S. (2021). Global prevalence of depressive and anxiety symptoms in children and adolescents during COVID-19: A meta-analysis. *JAMA Pediatrics, 175*(11), 1142-1150. https://doi.org/10.1001/jamapediatrics.2021.2482

Radloff, L. S. (1977). The CES-D scale: A self-report report depression scale for research in the general population. *Applied Psychological Measurement, 1*(3), 385-401. https://doi.org/10.1177/014662167700100306

Rea, M. M., Tompson, M. C., Miklowitz, D. J., Goldstein, M. J., Hwang, S., & Mintz, J. (2003). Family-focused treatment versus individual treatment for bipolar disorder: Results of a randomized clinical trial. *Journal of Consulting and Clinical Psychology, 71*(3), 482-492. https://doi.org/10.1037/0022-006X.71.3.482

Reinherz, H. Z., Giaconia, R. M., Lefkowitz, E. S., Pakiz, B., & Frost, A. K. (1993). Prevalence of psychiatric disorders in a community population of older adolescents. *Journal of the American Academy of Child & Adolescent Psychiatry, 32*(3), 369-377. https://doi.org/10.1097/00004583-199303000-00019

Restifo, K., & Bögels, S. (2009). Family processes in the development of youth depression: Translating the evidence to treatment. *Clinical Psychology Review, 29*(4), 294-316.

Roberts, R. E., & Chen, Y.-W. (1995). Depressive symptoms and suicidal ideation among Mexican-origin and Anglo adolescents. *Journal of the American Academy of Child & Adolescent Psychiatry, 34*(1), 81-90. https://doi.org/10.1097/00004583-199501000-00018

Roberts, R. E., Roberts, C. R., & Chen, Y. R. (1997). Ethnocultural differences in prevalence of adolescent depression. *American Journal of Community Psychology, 25*(1), 95-110. https://doi.org/10.1023/A:1024649925737

Robin, A. L., & Weisz, J. G. (1980). Criterion-related validity of behavioral and self-report measures of problem-solving communication skills in distressed and non-distressed parent-adolescent dyads. *Behavioral Assessment, 2*, 339-352.

Rohde, P., Lewinsohn, P. M., Klein, D. N., Seeley, J. R., & Gau, J. M. (2013). Key characteristics of major depressive disorder occurring in childhood, adolescence, emerging adulthood, and adulthood. *Clinical Psychological Science, 1*(1), 41-53. https://doi.org/10.1177/2167702612457599

Rothbart, M. K., Ahadi, S. A., & Evans, D. E. (2000). Temperament and personality: Origins and outcomes. *Journal of Personality and Social Psychology, 78*(1), 122-135. https://doi.org/10.1037/0022-3514.78.1.122

Rotheram-Borus, M. J., Piacentini, J., Miller, S., Graae, F., & Castro-Blanco, D. (1994). Brief cognitive-behavioral treatment for adolescent suicide attempters and their families. *Journal of the American Academy of Child & Adolescent Psychiatry, 33*(4), 508-517. https://doi.org/10.1097/00004583-199405000-00009

Ruch, D. A., Sheftall, A. H., Schlagbaum, P., Rausch, J., Campo, J. V., & Bridge, J. A. (2019). Trends in suicide among youth aged 10 to 19 years in the United States,

1975 to 2016. *JAMA Network Open, 2*(5), e193886. https://doi.org/10.1001/jamanetworkopen.2019.3886

Rudolph, K. D., Flynn, M., & Abaied, J. L. (2008). A developmental perspective on interpersonal theories of youth depression. In J. R. Z. Abela & B. L. Hankin (Eds.), *Handbook of depression in children and adolescents* (pp. 79–102). Guilford Press.

Rudolph, K. D., & Hammen, C. (1999). Age and gender as determinants of stress exposure, generation, and reactions in youngsters: A transactional perspective. *Child Development, 70*(3), 660–677. https://doi.org/10.1111/1467-8624.00048

Rush, A. J., Trivedi, M. H., Ibrahim, H. M., Carmody, T. J., Arnow, B., Klein, D. N., Markowitz, J. C., Ninan, P. T., Kornstein, S., Manber, R., Thase, M. E., Kocsis, J. H., & Keller, M. B. (2003). The 16-item Quick Inventory of Depressive Symptomatology (QIDS), clinician rating (QIDS-C), and self-report (QIDS-SR): A psychometric evaluation in patients with chronic major depression. *Biological Psychiatry, 54*(5), 573–583. https://doi.org/10.1016/S0006-3223(02)01866-8

Salk, R. H., Hyde, J. S., & Abramson, L. Y. (2017). Gender differences in depression in representative national samples: Meta-analyses of diagnoses and symptoms. *Psychological Bulletin, 143*(8), 783–822. https://doi.org/10.1037/bul0000102

Sanchez, A. L., Comer, J. S., & LaRoche, M. (2022). Enhancing the responsiveness of family-based CBT through culturally informed case conceptualization and treatment planning. *Cognitive and Behavioral Practice, 29*(4), 750–770. https://doi.org/10.1016/j.cbpra.2021.04.003

Sawyer, M. G., Reece, C. E., Sawyer, A. C. P., Johnson, S. E., & Lawrence, D. (2018). Has the prevalence of child and adolescent mental disorders in Australia changed between 1998 and 2013 to 2014? *Journal of the American Academy of Child & Adolescent Psychiatry, 57*(5), 343–350. https://doi.org/10.1016/j.jaac.2018.02.012

Shaffer, D., Fisher, P., Dulcan, M. K., & Davies, M. (1996). The NIMN Diagnostic Interview Schedule for Children version 2.3 (DISC-2.3): Description, acceptability, prevalence rates, and performance in the MECA study. *Journal of the American Academy of Child & Adolescent Psychiatry, 35*(7), 865–877.

Shaffer, D., Schwab-Stone, M., Fisher, P. W., Cohen, P., Placentini, J., Davies, M., Conners, C. K., & Regier, D. (1993). The Diagnostic Interview Schedule for Children – revised version (DISC-R): I Preparation, field testing, interrater reliability, and acceptability. *Journal of the American Academy of Child & Adolescent Psychiatry, 32*(3), 643–650. https://doi.org/10.1097/00004583-199305000-00023

Shanahan, L., Copeland, W. E., Costello, E. J., & Angold, A. (2011). Child-, adolescent- and young adult-onset depressions: Differential risk factors in development? *Psychological Medicine, 41*(11), 2265–2274. https://doi.org/10.1017/S0033291710000675

Shapero, B. G., Chai, X. J., Vangel, M., Biederman, J., Hoover, C. S., Whitfield-Gabrieli, S., Gabrieli, J., & Hirshfeld-Becker, D. R. (2019). Neural markers of depression risk predict the onset of depression. Psychiatry Research. *Neuroimaging, 285*, 31–39. https://doi.org/10.1016/j.pscychresns.2019.01.006

Sheeber, L., Hops, H., Alpert, A., Davis, B., & Andrews, J. (1997). Family support and conflict: Prospective relations to adolescent depression. *Journal of Abnormal Child Psychology, 25*(4), 333–344. https://doi.org/10.1023/A:1025768504415

Silverman, W. K., & Albano, A. M. (1996). *The Anxiety Disorders Interview Schedule for Children (ADIS-C/P)*. Psychological Corporation.

Simonoff, E., Pickles, A., Meyer, J. M., Silberg, J. L., Maes, H. H., Loeber, R., Rutter, M., Hewitt, J. K., & Eaves, L. J. (1997). The Virginia twin study of adolescent behavioral development: Influence of age, sex, and impairment on rates of disorder. *Archives of General Psychiatry, 54*(9), 801–808. https://doi.org/10.1001/archpsyc.1997.01830210039004

Southam-Gerow, M. A., & Prinstein, M. J. (2014). Evidence base updates: The evolution of the evaluation of psychological treatments for children and adolescents.

Journal of Clinical Child & Adolescent Psychology, 43(1), 1–6. https://doi.org/10.1080/15374416.2013.855128

Stice, E., Ragan, J., & Randall, P. (2004). Prospective relations between social support and depression: Differential direction of effects for parent and peer support? *Journal of Abnormal Psychology, 113*(1), 155–159. https://doi.org/10.1037/0021-843X.113.1.155

Stockmeier, C. A. (2003). Involvement of serotonin in depression: Evidence from postmortem and imaging studies of serotonin receptors and the serotonin transporter. *Journal of Psychiatric Research, 37*(5), 357–373. https://doi.org/10.1016/S0022-3956(03)00050-5

Tompson, M. C., Asarnow, J. R., Mintz, J., & Cantwell, D. P. (2015). Parental depression risk: Comparing youth with depression, attention deficit hyperactivity disorder and community controls. *Journal of Psychology & Psychotherapy, 5*(4), 1. https://doi.org/10.4172/2161-0487.1000193

Tompson, M. C., Boger, K. D., & Asarnow, J. R. (2012). Enhancing the developmental appropriateness of treatment for depression in youth: Integrating the family in treatment. *Child and Adolescent Psychiatric Clinics of North America, 21*(2), 345–384. https://doi.org/10.1016/j.chc.2012.01.003

Tompson, M. C., Langer, D. A., & Asarnow, J. R. (2020). Development and efficacy of a family-focused treatment for depression in childhood. *Journal of Affective Disorders, 276*, 686–695. https://doi.org/10.1016/j.jad.2020.06.057

Tompson, M. C., Langer, D. A., Hughes, J. L., & Asarnow, J. R. (2017). Family-focused treatment for childhood depression: Model and case illustrations. *Cognitive and Behavioral Practice, 24*(3), 269–287. https://doi.org/10.1016/j.cbpra.2016.06.003

Tompson, M. C., Pierre, C. B., Haber, F. M., Fogler, J. M., Groff, A. R., & Asarnow, J. R. (2007). Family-focused treatment for childhood-onset depressive disorders: Results of an open trial. *Clinical Child Psychology and Psychiatry, 12*(6), 403–420. https://doi.org/10.1177/1359104507078474

Tompson, M. C., Sugar, C. A., Langer, D. A., & Asarnow, J. R. (2017). A randomized clinical trial comparing family-focused treatment and individual supportive therapy for depression in childhood and early adolescence. *Journal of the American Academy of Child & Adolescent Psychiatry, 56*(6), 515–523. https://doi.org/10.1016/j.jaac.2017.03.018

Tompson, M. C., Swetlitz, C., & Asarnow, J. A. (2021). A family-based approach to the treatment of youth depression. In J. Allen, D. Hawes, & C. Essau (Eds.), *Family-based interventions for child and adolescent mental health* (pp. 87–99). Cambridge University Press.

Turner, J. E., & Cole, D. A. (1994). Developmental differences in cognitive diatheses for child depression. *Journal of Abnormal Child Psychology, 22*(1), 15–32. https://doi.org/10.1007/BF02169254

Twenge, J. M., Cooper, A. B., Joiner, T. E., Duffy, M. E., & Binau, S. G. (2019). *Age, period, and cohort trends in mood disorder indicators and suicide-related outcomes in a nationally representative dataset*, 2005–2017. *Journal of Abnormal Psychology, 128*(3), 185–199.

US Department of Health and Human Services. (2021). *U.S. surgeon general issues advisory on youth mental health crisis further exposed by COVID-19 pandemic*. https://www.hhs.gov/about/news/2021/12/07/us-surgeon-general-issues-advisory-on-youth-mental-health-crisis-further-exposed-by-covid-19-pandemic.html

Van Beveren, M. L., Mezulis, A., Wante, L., & Braet, C. (2019). Joint contributions of negative emotionality, positive emotionality, and effortful control on depressive symptoms in youth. *Journal of Clinical Child & Adolescent Psychology, 48*(1), 131–142. https://doi.org/10.1080/15374416.2016.1233499

Varni, J. W., Magnus, B., Stucky, B. D., Liu, Y., Quinn, H., Thissen, D., Gross, H. E., Huang, I.-C., & DeWalt, D. A. (2014). Psychometric properties of the PROMIS® pediatric scales: Precision, stability, and comparison of different scoring and administration options. *Quality of Life Research, 23*(4), 1233–1243. https://doi.org/10.1007/s11136-013-0544-0

Velez, C. N., Johnson, J., & Cohen, P. (1989). A longitudinal analysis of selected risk factors for childhood psychopathology. *Journal of the American Academy of Child & Adolescent Psychiatry, 28*(6), 861–864. https://doi.org/10.1097/00004583-198911000-00009

Weersing, V. R., Jeffreys, M., Do, M.-C. T., Schwartz, K. T. G., & Bolano, C. (2017). Evidence base update of psychosocial treatments for child and adolescent depression. *Journal of Clinical Child & Adolescent Psychology, 46*(1), 11–43. https://doi.org/10.1080/15374416.2016.1220310

Weissman, M. M., Gammon, G. D., John, K., Merikangas, K. R., Warner, V., Prusoff, B. A., & Sholomskas, D. (1987). Children of depressed parents: Increased psychopathology and early onset of major depression. *Archives of General Psychiatry, 44*(10), 847–853. https://doi.org/10.1001/archpsyc.1987.01800220009002

Weissman, M. M., Wolk, S., Goldstein, R. B., Moreau, D., Adams, P., Greenwald, S., Klier, C. M., Ryan, N. D., Dahl, R. E., & Wickramaratne, P. (1999). Depressed adolescents grown up. *JAMA, 281*(11), 1707–1713. https://doi.org/10.1001/jama.281.18.1707

Weller, E., Weller, R., Fristad, M., Rooney, M. T., & Schechter, J. (2000). Children's interview for psychiatric syndromes (ChIPS). *Journal of the American Academy of Child & Adolescent Psychiatry, 39*(1), 76–84. https://doi.org/10.1097/00004583-200001000-00019

Weller, R. A., Kapadia, P., Weller, E. B., Fristad, M., Lazaroff, L., & Preskorn, S. H. (1994). Psychopathology in families of children with major depressive disorders. *Journal of Affective Disorders, 31*(4), 247–252. https://doi.org/10.1016/0165-0327(94)90100-7

Wichstrøm, L., Berg-Nielsen, T. S., Angold, A., Egger, H. L., Solheim, E., & Sveen, T. H. (2012). Prevalence of psychiatric disorders in preschoolers. *Journal of Child Psychology and Psychiatry, 53*(6), 695–705.

World Health Organization (WHO). (1993). *The ICD-10 classification of mental and behavioural disorders: Diagnostic criteria for research*. https://www.who.int/publications/i/item/9241544228

Wyatt, L. C., Ung, T., Park, R., Kwon, S. C., & Trinh-Shevrin, C. (2015). Risk factors of suicide and depression among Asian American, Native Hawaiian, and Pacific Islander youth: A systematic literature review. *Journal of Health Care for the Poor and Underserved, 26*(2 Suppl), 191–237. https://doi.org/10.1353/hpu.2015.0059

Yard, E., Radhakrishnan, L., Ballesteros, M. F., Sheppard, M., Gates, A., Stain, Z., Hartnett, K., Kite-Powell, A., Rodgers, L., Adjemian, J., Ehlman, D. C., Holland, K., Idaikkadar, N., Ivey-Stephenson, A., Martinez, P., Law, R., & Stone, D. M. (2021, June 18). Emergency department visits for suspected suicide attempts among persons ages 12–25 years before and during the COVID-19 pandemic: United States, January 2019–May 2021. *Morbidity and Mortality Weekly Report, 70*(24), 888–894. https://www.cdc.gov/mmwr/volumes/70/wr/mm7024e1.htm

Zhang, J., Lam, S. P., Li, S. X., Liu, Y., Chan, J. W. Y., Chan, M. H. M., Ho, C. S., Li, A. M., & Wing, Y. K. (2018). Parental history of depression and higher basal salivary cortisol in unaffected child and adolescent offspring. *Journal of Affective Disorders, 234*, 207–213. https://doi.org/10.1016/j.jad.2018.02.086

Zisook, S., Lesser, I., Stewart, J. W., Wisniewski, S. R., Balasubramani, G. K., Fava, M., Gilmer, W. S., Dresselhaus, T. R., Thase, M. E., Nierenberg, A. A., Trivedi, M. H., & Rush, A. J. (2007). Effect of age at onset on the course of major depressive disorder. *American Journal of Psychiatry, 164*(10), 1539–1546. https://doi.org/10.1176/appi.ajp.2007.06101757

8 Appendix: Tools and Resources

The following materials for your book can be downloaded free of charge once you register on the Hogrefe website:

Appendix 1: FFT-CD Treatment Handouts
Handout 1   Thoughts, Feelings, Actions
Handout 2   Feelings and How We Act
Handout 3   Downward Spiral
Handout 4   Upward Spiral
Handout 5   Catching Upward Spirals
Handout 6   Saying What You Liked
Handout 7   Keeping Upward Spirals Going
Handout 8   Active Listening
Handout 9   Catching Downward Spirals
Handout 10   Saying What You Didn't Like
Handout 11   Stopping Downward Spirals
Handout 12   Fun Activities
Handout 13   Asking for What You Want
Handout 14   Fun Things to Do
Handout 15   Defining Problems
Handout 16   What's the Problem?
Handout 17   Emotional Thermometer
Handout 18   Solving Problems
Handout 19   Problem Solving Worksheet

Appendix 2: Supplementary Handouts
Symptoms of Depression
How People Get Symptoms of Depression
Mood Monitoring
Ideas for Fun Activities

Appendix 3: Games for Use With FFT-CD

Positive Feedback: Silly

Positive Feedback: Serious

Game Listening A

Game Listening B

Game Listening C

Negative Feedback: Silly

Negative Feedback: Serious

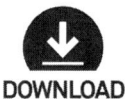

How to proceed:

1. Go to www.hgf.io/media and create a user account. If you already have one, please log in.

2. Go to **My supplementary materials** in your account dashboard and enter the code below. You will automatically be redirected to the download area, where you can access and download the supplementary materials.

Code: B-PQZBJD

To make sure you have permanent direct access to all the materials, we recommend that you download them and save them on your computer.

8. Appendix: Tools and Resources 101

Appendix 1: FFT-CD Treatment Handouts

This is a **preview** of the content that is available in the downloadable material of this book. Please see p. 99 for instructions on how to obtain the full-sized, printable PDF.

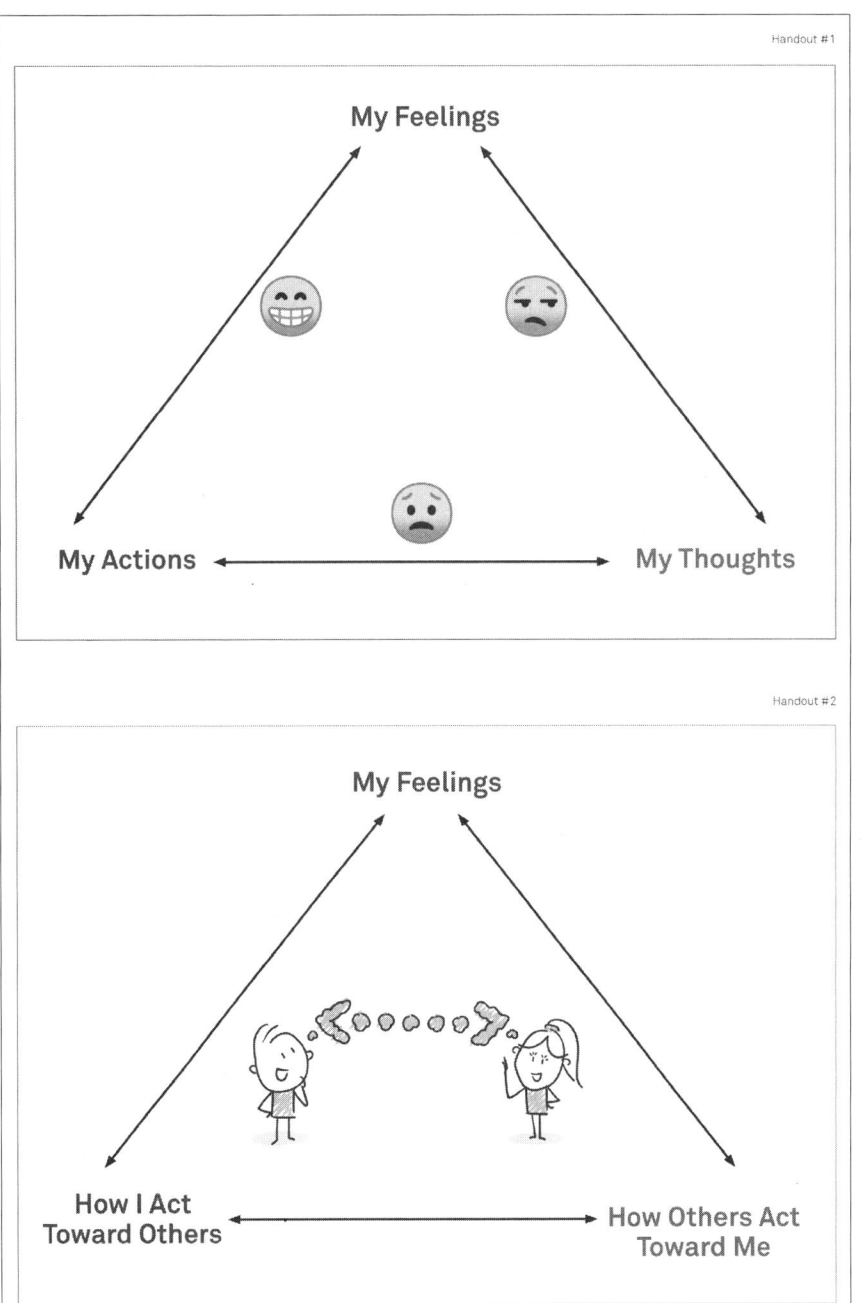

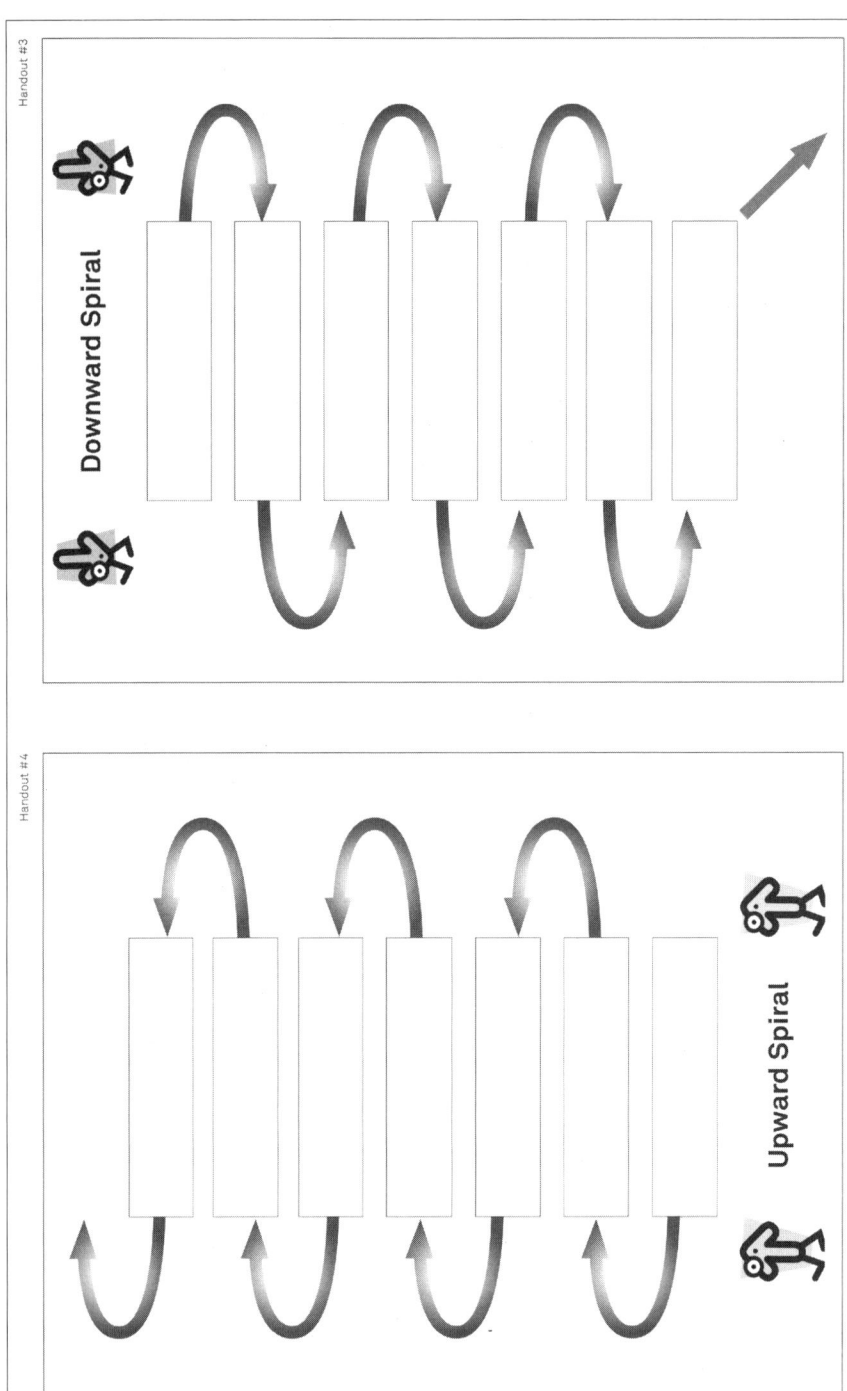

This is a **preview** of the content that is available in the downloadable material of this book. Please see p. 99 for instructions on how to obtain the full-sized, printable PDF.

8. Appendix: Tools and Resources

Handout #5

Catching Upward Spirals

Day of the week	Person who did something nice	What they did	How it made you feel
Monday			
Tuesday			
Wednesday			
Thursday			
Friday			
Saturday			
Sunday			

Examples

Looking Good	Being on Time	Helping at Home	Work in the Yard
Coming to Session	Having a Chat	Going to Work/School	Offering to Help
Making a Suggestion	Being Considerate	Going Out	Taking Medicine
Cooking Meals	Smiling	Doing Homework	

Handout #6

Saying What You Liked

- Look at the person

- Say exactly what they did that you liked

- Tell them how it made you feel

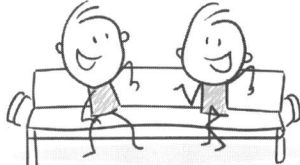

This is a **preview** of the content that is available in the downloadable material of this book. Please see p. 99 for instructions on how to obtain the full-sized, printable PDF.

Handout #7

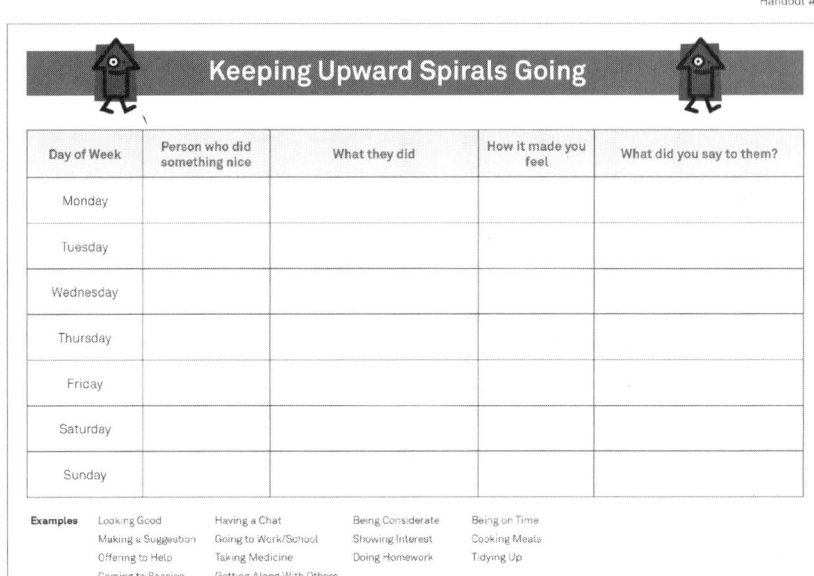

Keeping Upward Spirals Going

Day of Week	Person who did something nice	What they did	How it made you feel	What did you say to them?
Monday				
Tuesday				
Wednesday				
Thursday				
Friday				
Saturday				
Sunday				

Examples
Looking Good · Having a Chat · Being Considerate · Being on Time
Making a Suggestion · Going to Work/School · Showing Interest · Cooking Meals
Offering to Help · Taking Medicine · Doing Homework · Tidying Up
Coming to Session · Getting Along With Others

Handout #8

Active Listening

- Look at the person speaking

- Listen *carefully*

- Nod your head, say "uh-huh"

- Ask questions to clear it up

- Check out what you heard

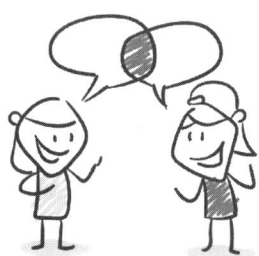

This is a **preview** of the content that is available in the downloadable material of this book. Please see p. 99 for instructions on how to obtain the full-sized, printable PDF.

8. Appendix: Tools and Resources

Handout #9

 **Catching Downward Spirals**

Day of Week	Person who did something you didn't like	What they did	How it made you feel
Monday			
Tuesday			
Wednesday			
Thursday			
Friday			
Saturday			
Sunday			

Examples
Mom picked me up late from school. It made me feel _____.
Bobby forgot to do his homework. It made me feel _____.
Jenny made a mess in the kitchen. It made me feel _____.
Dad yelled at me. It made me feel _____.

Handout #10

 Saying What You Didn't Like

- Look 'em in the eye
- Say exactly what bothered you
- Say how it made you feel
- What they can do in the future

1. No name-calling
2. No going on and on – be brief
3. Don't forget to be specific

This is a **preview** of the content that is available in the downloadable material of this book. Please see p. 99 for instructions on how to obtain the full-sized, printable PDF.

Stopping Downward Spirals

Handout #11

Day of week	Who did what you didn't like	What didn't you like	What would you rather they do	Did you?			
				Look 'em in the eye	Tell 'em what bothered you	Tell 'em how it made you feel	Tell 'em what they could do in the future
Example: Monday	Mom	She let my brother use my iPod	Ask me first if it is okay with me	✓	✓	✓	✓

Handout #12

Fun Activites

Fun things to do	Who do you like to do this with?				How often do you do this?	How much fun is it?
	Family	Friends	Alone	?		
1. Go to the movies		✓			Once a month	Really fun (7)
2. Play a board game	✓				Every Wednesday	5
3. Do arts & crafts			✓		Two times a week	6
4.						
5.						
6.						
7.						
8.						
9.						
10.						

How much fun is it?

1	2	3	4	5	6	7
Boring		A little fun		Pretty fun		Really fun

This is a **preview** of the content that is available in the downloadable material of this book. Please see p. 99 for instructions on how to obtain the full-sized, printable PDF.

8. Appendix: Tools and Resources

Handout #13

Asking For What You Want

- Look at the person

- Say exactly what you would like them to do

- Tell how it would make you feel

When asking for what you want, try saying ...
"I would like you to _____."
"I would appreciate it if you would _____."
"It's very important to me that you help _____."

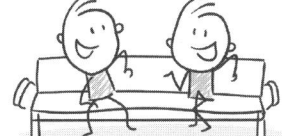

Handout #14

Fun Things to Do

Activity	Who's included?	When do we do this?	Did it happen?	How much fun was it?
1.				
2.				
3.				
4.				
5.				
6.				
7.				
8.				
9.				
10.				

How much fun was it?

1 — Boring 2 3 — A little fun 4 5 — Pretty fun 6 7 — Really fun

---

This is a **preview** of the content that is available in the downloadable material of this book. Please see p. 99 for instructions on how to obtain the full-sized, printable PDF.

Handout #15

Defining Problems

Rules of Problem Solving

- No name-calling or blaming
- Figure out who is involved
- Get all sides (everyone has their say)
- Be specific
- Keep it short and sweet

Remember ... how would you know it was solved?

Sometimes Problems Can't Be Solved:

- When they are way too big
- When they happened in the past
- When they are out of your control

Handout #16

What's the Problem?

Problem?	Who's included?	How often does it happen?	Emotional temperature
1.			
2.			
3.			
4.			
5.			
6.			
7.			

This is a **preview** of the content that is available in the downloadable material of this book. Please see p. 99 for instructions on how to obtain the full-sized, printable PDF.

8. Appendix: Tools and Resources   109

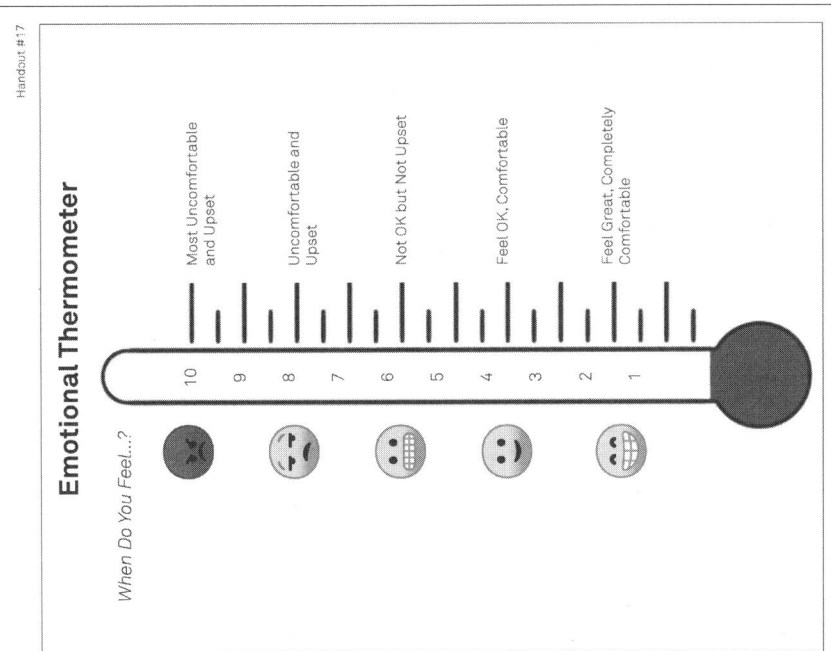

Handout #17

Emotional Thermometer

- Most Uncomfortable and Upset
- Uncomfortable and Upset
- Not OK but Not Upset
- Feel OK, Comfortable
- Feel Great, Completely Comfortable

When Do You Feel...?

Handout #18

Solving Problems

- Agree on the problem
- Come up with some ideas to solve it
- Discuss pluses and minuses of each
- Agree on the best plan
- Carry out the plan
- Decide if it worked and praise everyone for their efforts

This is a **preview** of the content that is available in the downloadable material of this book. Please see p. 99 for instructions on how to obtain the full-sized, printable PDF.

Handout #19

Problem Solving Worksheet

Step 1 Define "What's the Problem?" Talk. Listen. Ask questions. Get everybody's opinion.

_____
_____

Step 2 List all possible solutions. "Brainstorm" – put down all ideas, even bad ones. Get everybody to come up with at least one idea. DO NOT EVALUATE ANY SOLUTION AT THIS POINT.

_____
_____

Step 3 Discuss and list all pluses and minuses of each possible solution.

Pluses   Minuses

_____   _____
_____   _____
_____   _____
_____   _____

Step 4 Choose the best possible solution and list here. (May be a combination of possible solutions)

_____
_____

Step 5 Plan how to carry out the chosen solution, AND set a date to start. Date: _____

- Specifically decide who will do what. List here.

  _____
  _____

- Decide what things will be needed, list here, and obtain them.

  _____

- List here what could go wrong and figure out how to deal with it.

  _____
  _____

- Practice the solution.
- DO IT! (On schedule)

Step 6 Review the solution and give praise to everyone who worked it out.

_____

Step 7 If unsuccessful, go back to Step 1 and try again. Solutions often aren't perfect the first time, so don't get discouraged!

This is a **preview** of the content that is available in the downloadable material of this book. Please see p. 99 for instructions on how to obtain the full-sized, printable PDF.

8. Appendix: Tools and Resources

Appendix 2: Supplementary Handouts

This is a **preview** of the content that is available in the downloadable material of this book. Please see p. 99 for instructions on how to obtain the full-sized, printable PDF.

Symptoms of Depression

- Low mood, sadness, feeling "down in the dumps," feel like crying
- Irritability, anger or "grumpiness"
- More hungry or less hungry than usual; gaining or losing weight
- Sleeping too much or too little
- Low energy, tiredness
- Little interest in doing things or don't enjoy doing things
- Doing fewer things; withdrawing from others
- Thoughts of hurting or killing yourself
- Having a hard time thinking and concentrating
- Feeling worthless and really guilty about things

How Do People Get Symptoms of Depression?

- Depression runs in families
- People may have a genetic predisposition to get depressed (same is true for other kinds of problems, like heart disease)
- People may have a physical tendency (in the brain) toward getting depressed
- Life stress and changes can lead to depression (even *good* changes are hard to deal with!)
- Negative thinking, when it happens a lot, can lead to depression

Mood Monitoring

Date	Time	Where were you?	Who were you with?	What were you doing?	How did you feel?	How strong was that feeling from 0 (not strong) to 8 (the strongest)?	What did you do to feel better?

Ideas For Fun Activities

Circle activities that would be fun for you, and write some of your own!

Going to museums/aquariums/zoos	Drawing outside with chalk	Blowing bubbles	Listening to music
Playing jump-rope	Going to plays/concerts	Working with others in a team	Rearranging/redecorating the house
Singing/dancing	Taking a long bath or shower	Watching/playing sports	Doing arts and crafts
Starting a new project	Thinking about something good in the future	Learning something new	Being with animals
Solving a puzzle or crossword	Flying a kite	Going to church/temple/mosque	Volunteering
Talking on the phone	Going to school-related events/fieldtrips	Spending time with family	Going to the movies
Planning/taking fun trips	Doing things with younger siblings	Making new/special food	Playing games with others
Going for a walk/playing outside	Meditating or doing yoga	Biking/rollerblading	Playing computer/video games
Being outdoors (park, beach, doing outdoors work)	Planning or organizing something	Writing cards, letters, or notes for someone	Reading a book/magazine/newspaper
Wearing clothes I like/playing dress-up	• _____ • _____	• _____ • _____	• _____ • _____

This is a **preview** of the content that is available in the downloadable material of this book. Please see p. 99 for instructions on how to obtain the full-sized, printable PDF.

Appendix 3: Games for Use With FFT-CD

> This is a **preview** of the content that is available in the downloadable material of this book. Please see p. 99 for instructions on how to obtain the full-sized, printable PDF.

Positive Feedback: Silly

1. I couldn't believe it when you ate ten hamburgers for breakfast. That made me feel _____
2. When we built that upside down snowman together, it made me feel _____
3. When we went to the movies wearing our bathing suits and swim goggles, it made me feel _____
4. I liked it when you brought home that tiger as a pet. It made me feel _____
5. I really like the way you stand on your head and stick your tongue out. It makes me feel _____
6. I liked it when you helped the chicken cross the road. It made me feel _____ (But why did he do it?)
7. I liked it when you gave me a piggy-back ride to school. It made me feel _____
8. I liked it when you wore a wig with spiked silver hair. It made me feel _____
9. I liked it when you dressed up as a monkey to go rollerblading. That made me feel _____
10. I liked it when you made me a pickle, jelly, and mustard sandwich. It made me feel _____
11. I liked it when you went bowling in your pajamas. It made me feel _____
12. It was interesting when you wore your socks on your hands and your gloves on your feet. It made me feel _____
13. I liked it when you brought that elephant home. It made me feel _____
14. I was glad when you dressed in your clown suit and played your drums. It made me feel _____
15. I liked it when you gave me the flowers made out of cheese-whiz. It made me feel _____
16. I enjoyed going to see the monkeys who sing in a barbershop quartet with you. It made me feel _____
17. When you took me to school in a purple and green polka dotted Corvette, it made me feel _____
18. I liked it when we built an airplane out of Legos and then flew it to Australia together. It made me feel _____

Positive Feedback: Serious

1. When I got a good grade on that test and you took me to get ice cream to celebrate it made me feel _____
2. I appreciate it when you say things to make me laugh. It makes me feel _____
3. When you took me to the park and we played catch, it made me feel _____
4. I liked it when you let me borrow your favorite CD. It made me feel _____
5. When you took me to the hockey game, it made me feel _____
6. When we went fishing together, it made me feel _____
7. When we had a four-hour long checkers tournament, it made me feel _____
8. Last night you made my favorite dinner. That made me feel _____
9. I appreciate it when you give me a hug. It makes me feel _____
10. I liked it when you invited me to play video games with you. It made me feel _____
11. When I got home from school and you asked me how my day was, it made me feel _____
12. I liked it when you helped me out. It made me feel _____
13. When you took me to the soccer game last week, it made me feel _____
14. I liked it when you took me to the library to take out some books, it made me feel _____
15. I liked it when you rented my favorite movie and we popped popcorn. That made me feel _____
16. It was good that you sold so many Girl Scout cookies. It made me feel _____
17. It was great that you helped me with dinner. It made me feel _____
18. I liked it when we read a book together before bed. It made me feel _____
19. When you told me that you love me, it made me feel _____
20. I liked it when you told me that you were proud of me. It made me feel _____

Game Listening B

Active listening with affect (role-playing others)

1. Bobby's mom said she would take him to get ice cream, but then something came up and she couldn't. How do you think Bobby felt?
2. Mary just failed her third test in a row. If you were Mary, what would you be thinking and feeling?
3. Jack just started his first day at a new school, where he doesn't know anybody. If you were Jack, how do you think you would feel?
4. Classmates teased Sally for having trouble reading in class. How do you think Sally felt?
5. Rachel got the lead in the school play. How do you think Rachel feels?
6. Katie's teacher just told her that the project she turned in was her best work yet. If you were Katie, how would you feel?
7. Tom just won tickets to see his favorite band in concert. How do you think Tom feels?
8. Tim's teacher just caught him cheating on a test. If you were Tim, what would you be thinking and feeling?
9. Laura was late to her softball game, so her coach made her sit out the whole time. How do you think Laura felt?
10. John hurt his ankle and had to wear a cast to school for a month. How do you think he felt?
11. Kim accidently broke her mother's favorite vase while playing soccer inside the house. How do you think Kim felt while waiting for her mother to come home from work?
12. Ashley spent the whole day thinking no one remembered her birthday, but at night her friends surprised her with a big party. How do you think her thoughts and feelings changed before and after the surprise?

Game Listening A

Active listening with content only (no affect)

1. Describe how you would make a peanut butter and jelly sandwich, with every step that's involved.
2. Describe how you get ready for bed at night (brushing teeth, putting pajamas on, reading in bed, etc).
3. If you got to go to Disney World for one day, talk about what you would do.
4. Talk about what happens when you go out to your favorite place to eat.
5. Describe what you do when you go to the library or the park.
6. If you could spend a Saturday afternoon doing anything you wanted, describe what you would do and who you would spend it with.
7. Describe what you do during your favorite class in school.
8. Describe an activity you like to do with your family.
9. Talk about something you like to do when you are outside.
10. Describe something you love to do in the summer.
11. Talk about something you like to do on your favorite holiday.
12. If you could bring anything to school for "show and tell," what would you bring?
13. Describe your "getting ready for school" routine.

This is a **preview** of the content that is available in the downloadable material of this book. Please see p. 99 for instructions on how to obtain the full-sized, printable PDF.

Negative Feedback: Silly

1. I don't want you to stand on your head for five hours. It makes me feel _____. Next time, just stand on your head for an hour.
2. I would rather if you did not walk on the ceiling with your shoes on. It makes me feel _____. Next time, could you take your shoes off?
3. I would rather if you didn't put your face in the cereal. It makes me feel _____. Next time, eat your cereal with a spoon.
4. I don't like it when you drool on my pillow. It makes me feel _____. Next time, I would rather you slept on your own pillow.
5. I would rather you didn't fall asleep on top of the washing machine. It makes me feel _____. Next time, please try to sleep on the bed or couch.
6. I don't like it when you throw Brussels sprouts at dad; it makes me feel _____. Next time, tell him what he is doing that you don't like.
7. I would rather if you didn't eat the dog food. It makes me feel _____. Next time please eat the lasagna.
8. I don't like it when you put the dog in the dishwasher. It makes me feel _____. Next time wash him with the hose.
9. I would rather you did not eat your homework. It makes me feel _____. Next time, just put it in your book bag when you are done.
10. I don't like it when your dinosaur eats off the table. It makes me feel _____. Next time, feed the dinosaur outside.
11. I don't like it when you will only talk to me in Pig-Latin. It makes me feel _____. Next time please try to talk to me in a language I understand.
12. I don't like it when you come into my room and paint the walls purple. It makes me feel _____. Next time, please ask my permission to enter and change my space.
13. I don't like it when you expect me to have X-ray vision and are angry when I don't. It makes me feel _____. Next time, please try to accept my merely human capabilities.
14. I would rather you didn't leave your stuffed gerbils all around the house. It makes me feel _____. Next time, please put them in their stuffed gerbil cage.
15. I don't like it when you don't take care of your pet armadillo. It makes me feel _____. Next time, please remember to feed him and take him for his daily walk.
16. I don't like it when you complain about having to pick me up from Neptune. It makes me feel _____. Next time, please talk to me about what I can do to make things easier. I know it's a lot of work, but I have to be there for the interplanetary soccer game!

Game Listening C

Active listening with affect (about self)

1. Describe your least favorite food. What about it grosses you out?
2. Talk about a time when you saw something beautiful.
3. Describe when you smelled something really good.
4. Talk about a time when you were really frustrated.
5. Tell someone about a time when you were really excited for something.
6. Describe something that makes you really mad.
7. Describe a time when you felt really nervous or anxious about something.
8. Describe a time when you felt really scared.
9. Describe a time when you felt lonely.
10. What is one of your favorite songs, and how does it make you feel when you listen to it?
11. Describe a time when you felt really disappointed about something.
12. Talk about a time when you felt you were treated unfairly.
13. Describe something you have done that made you feel proud of yourself.
14. Talk about a time in which you were patient and understanding, even though it might have been difficult.

Negative Feedback: Serious

1. When you leave your muddy boots in the hallway, it makes me feel _____. Next time it would be nice if you left them outside.

2. I don't like it when you bump into me. It makes me feel _____. Next time, walk around me.

3. I don't like it when we have downward spirals. It makes me feel _____. Next time, let's plan a fun activity.

4. I don't like it when you let others play with my Game Boy without my permission. It makes me feel _____. Next time please ask my permission first.

5. I don't want you to leave the dishes in the sink until the end of the night. It makes me feel _____. Next time please wash them before 8 p.m.

6. I don't like it when you say you will play Scrabble with me and then don't. It makes me feel _____. Next time please do what you promised or talk to me about why you can't.

7. I don't like it when you yell at me. It makes me feel _____. Next time, please try to talk to me calmly.

8. I would rather you do your homework on time. When you don't, it makes me feel _____. Next time, please do it so that I don't have to keep nagging you.

17. I don't like it when you spend all your time working on your novel about French finger-painting. It makes me feel _____. Next time, can we please plan to spend some time doing an activity together?

18. I don't like it when you insist on eating only orange-colored food. It makes me feel _____. Next time, please try some other colored foods with the orange food.

19. I don't like it when you arrive home an hour late from water skiing with your friends. It makes me feel _____. Next time, please try to be on time or to call.

20. I don't like it when you criticize everything about the way I ride my unicycle. It makes me feel _____. Next time, please include some positive comments (like how my balance is improving) with the negative.

21. I don't like it when you won't tell me what went wrong during your expedition to the North Pole to see hyenas. It makes me feel _____. Next time, please try to talk to me.

22. I would rather that you tried harder in your classes, especially your "Fluffernutter Snowboarding" class. Your low effort makes me feel _____. Next time, please try harder and let me know how I can help you do better.

23. I don't like it when you yell at me for things like mixing up the cat and fish magnets on the refrigerator (the cats might eat the fish if they are stuck next to each other!). It makes me feel _____. Next time, please try to talk to me calmly about it and also tell me if there is something else bigger that is bothering you.

24. I don't like it when you move my collection of rubber band balls without telling me. It makes me feel _____. Next time, please talk to me before moving my things.

25. I would rather you didn't talk about my fear of red and purple striped squirrels with lots of people. It makes me feel _____. Next time, please keep these things private.

26. I would rather you didn't hang all of your furniture upside down from the ceiling. It makes me feel _____. Next time, please leave some of it on the floor – it is easier to use that way.

This is a **preview** of the content that is available in the downloadable material of this book. Please see p. 99 for instructions on how to obtain the full-sized, printable PDF.

Peer Commentaries

Dr. Tompson, an experienced clinician and nationally known researcher, provides in this book an up-to-date look at family-focused treatment for childhood depression (FFT-CD). She is the ideal person to do so given that she had a pivotal role in the development and formal testing of FFT-CD! A family-focused treatment approach is particularly appropriate when the patients are young school-aged children. But how will FFT-CD enable the clinician to resolve the complaints of depressed children and the accompanying family dysfunction? Dr. Tompson explains that skill building or skill enhancement (e. g., improving parent–child communication, developing more efficient problem-solving approaches) is the path to recovery. Thus, FFT-CD emphasizes functioning and uses modules to organize skill-focused tasks for the child and the family. For example, various skills come into play when the goal is to interrupt the "downward negative spiral" of depression that results from the interactions of the depressed child and family members. Another defining feature of FFT-CD is the flexible application of treatment components. The clinician has considerable leeway in which order and how the modules are implemented, the number of child-only vs. parents-only vs. family sessions, and how the recommended 12 to 15 sessions are distributed across treatment modules.

Case vignettes bring alive the process of implementing FFT-CD and document the flexibility of this intervention in the face of divergent patient needs and variable resources. Clinicians will especially appreciate the examples of how to define problematic concepts and the many "potential conversations," which illustrate how a therapist can engage a patient to implement new directions and tasks. As further aids, at the end of the book, readers will find downloadable tools such as hand-outs, illustrations, and games. For readers who wish to know more about childhood depression, the book reviews diagnostic criteria and up-to-date information about its key features such as course and outcome, presumed risk factors, and conceptual and treatment models. All-in-all, this book is a practical, useful, and accessible guide for therapists who seek to help depressed young school-age children and their families via a family-focused treatment approach.

Maria Kovacs, PhD, Distinguished Professor of Psychiatry, University of Pittsburgh School of Medicine, Pittsburgh, PA

This book is an extremely timely and state-of-the-art resource for any clinician seeking a comprehensive and user-friendly guide to the nature, assessment, and treatment of childhood depression. Written by one of the world's premier experts in childhood depression, this text helps readers understand why a developmentally informed, evidence-based, family-focused treatment approach is an indispensable tool for strengthening and supporting children with depression and their families. The inclusion of step-by-step descriptions of how to implement the treatment intervention, combined with illustrative case examples, will equip clinicians with powerful tools for helping youth return to healthier functioning during a critical period of development. The additional resources, games, and therapy handouts make this much more than a book – it is an essential tool for anyone working with depressed children and their families, and I highly recommend it!

Donna B. Pincus, PhD, CAS Feld Family Professor of Teaching Excellence, Department of Psychological and Brain Sciences, Boston University, MA

This thoughtful volume describes an excellent empirically validated, family-centered approach to treating depression in school-aged children developed by the author and her colleagues and outlines how to carry out therapy, session by session. It also presents the theoretical framework guiding the work and describes the impressive empirical research on which it is based. It is rich in clinical wisdom and insight and will provide excellent guidance to those wanting to use this approach. More generally it provides a valuable resource for those interested in depression in children and how to treat it.

William R. Beardslee, MD, Director, Baer Prevention Initiatives, Boston Children's Hospital, Boston, MA

The bad news is that childhood depression is on the rise. The good news is that Dr. Tompson has built upon her expertise as a childhood depression researcher, clinician, and educator to create an invaluable resource for clinicians. I highly recommend this book to all therapists who work with depressed children!

Mary A. Fristad, PhD, ABPP, Director, Academic Affairs and Research Development at Nationwide Children's Hospital Big Lots Behavioral Health Services, Columbus, OH; Emerita Professor, The Ohio State University, Columbus, OH

Advances in Psychotherapy – Evidence-Based Practice

Developed and edited with the support of the Society of Clinical Psychology (APA Division 12)

Editor-in-chief
Danny Wedding, PhD, MPH

Associate editors
Jonathan S. Comer, PhD
Linda Carter Sobell, PhD, ABPP
Kenneth E. Freedland, PhD
J. Kim Penberthy, PhD, ABPP

- *Practice-oriented*
- *Evidence-based*
- *Expert authors*
- *Easy-to-read*
- *Compact*
- *Cost-effective*

Latest releases

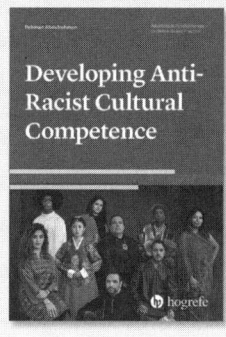

Volume 53

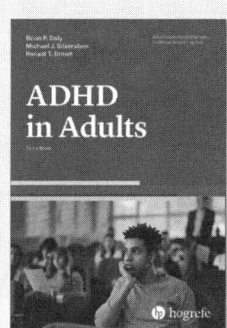

Volume 35

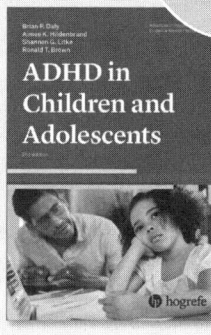

Volume 33

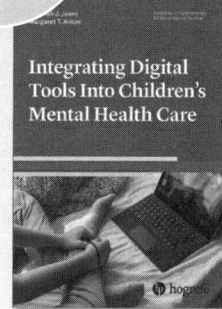

Volume 52

www.hogrefe.com/apt

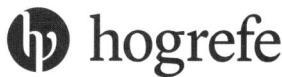

Advances in Psychotherapy – Evidence-Based Practice

All volumes of the series at a glance

Affirmative Counseling for Transgender and Gender Diverse Clients (Vol. 45)
Alcohol Use Disorders (Vol. 10)
Alzheimer's Disease and Dementia (Vol. 38)
ADHD in Adults, 2nd ed., (Vol. 35)
ADHD in Children and Adolescents, 2nd. ed., (Vol. 33)
Autism Spectrum Disorder (Vol. 29)
Binge Drinking and Alcohol Misuse Among College Students and Young Adults (Vol. 32)
Bipolar Disorder (Vol. 1, 2nd ed.)
Body Dysmorphic Disorder (Vol. 44)
Childhood Maltreatment (Vol. 4, 2nd ed.)
Childhood Obesity (Vol. 39)
Chronic Illness in Children and Adolescents (Vol. 9)
Chronic Pain (Vol. 11)
Depression (Vol. 18)
Developing Anti-Racist Cultural Competence (Vol. 53)
Eating Disorders (Vol. 13)
Elimination Disorders in Children and Adolescents (Vol. 16)
Family Caregiver Distress (Vol. 50)
Generalized Anxiety Disorder (Vol. 24)
Growing Up with Domestic Violence (Vol. 23)
Harm Reduction Treatment for Substance Use (Vol. 49)
Headache (Vol. 30)
Heart Disease (Vol. 2)
Hoarding Disorder (Vol. 40)
Hypochondriasis and Health Anxiety (Vol. 19)
Insomnia (Vol. 42)
Integrating Digital Tools into Children's Mental Health Care (Vol. 52)
Internet Addiction (Vol. 41)
Language Disorders in Children and Adolescents (Vol. 28)
Mindfulness (Vol. 37)
Multiple Sclerosis (Vol. 36)
Nicotine and Tobacco Dependence (Vol. 21)
Nonsuicidal Self-Injury (Vol. 22)
Obsessive-Compulsive Disorder in Adults (Vol. 31)
Occupational Stress (Vol. 51)
Persistent Depressive Disorders (Vol. 43)
Phobic and Anxiety Disorders in Children and Adolescents (Vol. 27)
Problem and Pathological Gambling (Vol. 8)
Psychological Approaches to Cancer Care (Vol. 46)
Public Health Tools for Practicing Psychologists (Vol. 20)
Sexual Dysfunction in Women (Vol. 25)
Sexual Dysfunction in Men (Vol. 26)
Sexual Violence (Vol. 17)
Social Anxiety Disorder (Vol. 12)
Substance Use Problems (Vol. 15, 2nd ed.)
Suicidal Behavior (Vol. 14, 2nd ed.)
The Schizophrenia Spectrum (Vol. 5, 2nd ed.)
Time-Out in Child Behavior Management (Vol. 48)
Treating Victims of Mass Disaster and Terrorism (Vol. 6)
Women and Drinking: Preventing Alcohol-Exposed Pregnancies (Vol. 34)

Prices: US $29.80 / € 24.95 per volume. Standing order price US $24.80 / € 19.95 per volume (minimum 4 successive volumes) + postage & handling. Special rates for APA Division 12 and Division 42 members

www.hogrefe.com/apt

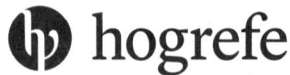